Home
Birth

Home Birth

An Invitation and a Guide

ALICE GILGOFF

BERGIN & GARVEY PUBLISHERS, INC.
MASSACHUSETTS

To Henry

First published in 1989 by
Bergin & Garvey Publishers, Inc.
670 Amherst Road
Granby, Massachusetts 01033

9   987654321

Printed in the United States of America

Library of Congress Cataloging-in-Publication Data

Gilgoff, Alice.
*   Home birth : an invitation and a guide / Alice Gilgoff.*
*   p.   cm.*
*   Bibliography: p.*
*   Includes index.*
*   ISBN 0–89789–179–1 (alk. paper) : $39.95.*
*   ISBN 0–89789–178–3 (pbk.: alk. paper) : $10.95*
*   1. Childbirth at home. I. Title.*
*   RG652.G54   1988*
*   618.4—dc19   88–27611*
*   CIP*

COVER PHOTOGRAPH: Byron Greatorex/Three Dragons
COVER DESIGN: Sue Katz/Graphic Design

Contents

Preface

So much has happened in the last ten years in the childbirth reform movement. The good news is that there are a lot more home births. The bad news is that the medical establishment is fighting even harder to stop them. Doctors and midwives have been harassed out of practice and parents have had home born babies snatched from their arms by government social service agencies supposedly interested in the child's welfare. And the alternative— hospital birth—is not immune to upheaval and conflict either. There may be more birthing rooms, but how often do they get used? With obstetricians practicing defensive medicine because of fear of malpractice suits, the cesarean rate has skyrocketed to more than 30 percent at some large teaching hospitals. It is almost as if this prediction ten years ago by a home birth physician is coming true: that some parents are being forced to choose between a normal birth in the home and a surgical delivery at the hospital.

But let's get back to the good news—home births are increasing. The topic has come out of the closet and onto the kitchen table.

Newspapers publish pleasant stories about a daughter of the famous Kennedy clan having one, and the psychiatrist writing the
afterword to Bill Cosby's *Fatherhood* casually refers to childbirth
"in the hospital, birthing center, or attended at home. . . ."

Still, an increase in numbers of births or amount of media exposure cannot erase the reality of the tension and conflict so many
parents are made to feel when they choose home birth. Warren
Pearse, while executive director of the American College of Obstetricians and Gynecologists, stated that home birth was child
abuse. Some legislators thought this was a mandate from the powerful medical lobby and took steps to enact Pearse's statement into
law. How does home birth increase in spite of such pressure? Because parents, knowing that larger issues of personal freedom and
control are involved, focus their attention on their priority—that
baby! And parents always act in the best interests of their children.
The challenge to make the best decision in the best interests of
the family and the new baby will always remain.

For their help along the way, I would like to thank Martin Kelly,
Vivian and Ralph McCraw, Beth Kava, Neil and Carol Offen, Dave
Zinman, Ken Gross, Theron Raines, Martha Habert, Carolyn
Hayes, Elaine Frey, Thelma and Russell Kottek, Diana Friedman,
Ruth Cohen, Lynn Richards, Jim Bergin, Ann Gross, Ilana Stein,
Michele Kaplan, Stephanie Goldstone, Marilyn Wecksell, and
Sally Mendelsohn.

For teaching me what I needed to know about love, Hugh Lorin,
Jon Noah, Matthew Dylan, Julie Ariane, and Joseph Kottek.

CHAPTER 1

"Their Way"

My first pregnancy was unplanned, and being new in a small community, my first difficulty was finding the right type of doctor to examine me. I finally located the chief of obstetrics and gynecology at the town's only hospital. After he told me I was pregnant, I told him I was interested in an unmedicated delivery. By his reaction, I could tell I wouldn't get his cooperation, and that to accomplish a natural birth, I'd be pretty much on my own.

The only birth book I found in the only local library was an old copy of *Childbirth Without Fear* by Grantly Dick-Read. At the time, Read's approach seemed too spiritual for me, but the one lesson I learned was that in order for anything like his method to work I had to have the support of my doctor.

I wrote the doctor I had seen a letter, telling him I could no longer be his patient and explaining why. And then the panic set in. Here I was, new in town, pregnant for the first time, and *not under a doctor's care*. What if I suddenly started to bleed? Images

1

of unknown tragedies that befell pregnant women ran through my mind.

I began frantic searches through telephone directories and called the medical societies and health departments in my county and the neighboring county. No one seemed to know or care about a doctor who supported natural childbirth. Each person I spoke to told me she could tell me the name of a doctor in my community and I could discuss it with him. But I had already seen the best my community had to offer.

So I went back to the phone books. I was becoming desperate. I looked up words like "Pregnancy," "Maternity," and "Babies." Then I tried fatter directories, from the closest big city. In the Manhattan book I found something under "Maternity." The listing was the Maternity Center Association, and the woman on the phone was the first person I had spoken to who knew what I was talking about. She even gave me the name of a doctor located a little less than thirty miles from me.

The doctor turned out to be knowledgeable, understanding, kind, and so paternalistic he seemed to feel that not only should every woman become a mother but the more "naturally" she did things the better mother she became. Strangely, this met my needs. He was the first person to mention Lamaze and La Leche League to me and to put me in touch with what each had to offer, childbirth preparation classes and instruction in breastfeeding. Whole new worlds began to open up for me. I felt confidence, fear, longing, wonderment, curiosity, and importance all at once. A new way of existence was revealed for me.

At the small suburban hospital, where husbands still were not allowed in the delivery room, this good doctor was supportive during labor, unlike the nurse who, during a strong contraction, pulled a pillow out from under me, gazed at some blood on it, and commented, "Childbirth is such a messy affair." In the delivery room, I pushed out a healthy eight-pound boy, without receiving an episiotomy (surgical cut to extend the vagina) or medication from the doctor. At my request, he even ordered a shocked nurse to hand me the baby to breastfeed on the delivery table.

I stayed at the hospital for three and a half days. I was not permitted to take a shower for thirty-six hours because I had given birth at 12:24 A.M., when the day was new, and the hospital rule was that a mother couldn't shower on the day she had given birth.

I couldn't eat for seven hours because I had to wait until the next scheduled meal. I received the baby to feed at four-hour intervals, although he wanted to nurse sooner. I bottlefed the baby a solution of 5 percent glucose in water, although this solution may be harmful to a newborn infant. But I didn't know any better. I just knew enough to know that I had been very lucky. I had set three standards for this birth—no drugs, no episiotomy, and nursing on the delivery table—and not only had I survived intact, but I had gotten the things I wanted, too.

When I became pregnant the second time it was two years later and I was in another community, closer to the big city. Lots of hospitals there were allowing husbands in the delivery room. My circle of child-bearing friends was seeking out doctors who did episiotomies for medical reasons only, not routinely, the kind of doctors who might let the baby nurse on the delivery table. Although I had already enjoyed these rights, I went to see a doctor whose name was mentioned more than once among my circle of friends, to find out what else he would offer. Yes, it was true an episiotomy might not be necessary but, no, the mother could not nurse on the delivery table as soon as the baby was born—the mother could nurse only in the wheelchair in which she sat after she got off the delivery table. The doctor was very rigid about this. When he delivered my friend's baby, six months before mine was to be born, the afterbirth did not come out soon enough following the baby. The doctor was impatient. Perhaps, my friend suggested, if she could have the baby now, breastfeeding would stimulate the uterus to contract, thereby expelling the placenta. But, no, nursing was for the wheelchair. He began to pull on the placenta, causing my friend to experience more pain than she had during her labor. The doctor warned her she would be "knocked out" with medication if she didn't calm down. He tugged some more. The placenta came out, in three parts.

My own falling-out with this doctor was not about placentas, but money. He wanted a large deposit by the second visit and payment in full by the eighth month. I told him if I were expecting a couch I wouldn't be required to pay in full two months before the delivery date. And weren't we dealing with human beings, not furniture? "I have been in practice since long before you were born, young lady," he began. Once more, I was without a doctor.

Several new names were suggested to me. My requirements for

a doctor were now even higher. If I had had some perspective then, I could have seen that I was heading in a certain direction where clashes had to occur. It took until my fifth month to find a doctor who agreed that it was not medically necessary for me to have an enema, a shave, or an episiotomy. Also, I could nurse on the delivery table—and go home two hours after birth if the baby and I were in good health.

I was ecstatic until, after labor began, I walked into the hospital and found that my doctor was not there yet. The resident who examined me ordered an enema and shave. No, I told him, my doctor and I had agreed this was not medically necessary. The resident was sorry, he could not possibly do as I wished. I was sorry, I could not possibly do as he wished. I asked him for the medical reasons. He could think of none for the shave. But the enema, he said, might have a therapeutic value in shaking up my labor since my bag of waters had broken a number of hours before and my contractions, once five minutes apart, had now come to a halt. So we compromised. He won on the enema, and I won on the shave. I don't know how he felt, but I was depressed. I had had certain expectations, I had been in the hospital less than twenty minutes, and already I had had to make compromises. (It would take me years to realize that the very fact of my labor coming to a halt was probably related to my arrival at the hospital in the first place.)

The resident never tested the therapeutic value of the enema. As soon as I was out of the bathroom I heard him consulting by phone with my doctor, and they agreed to adminster *Pitocin* (oxytocin), a drug for stimulating uterine contractions. I was given the drug in tablet form. Every twenty minutes a nurse placed two more tablets on my gums and the "Pit" was absorbed through my cheeks into my bloodstream. By the time my real doctor arrived I was promising myself to refuse the next two tablets. The medication was causing strong contractions to come in such rapid succession that it was extremely difficult, even with well-practiced breathing exercises, to control their effect. I never did stop breathing and scream out, but the force of the contractions was nearly overwhelming. Comparing them to my first labor I could see how unnatural they were and how close I kept coming to losing control.

When my doctor arrived, he joked that I'd "better hurry up" because he had a seven o'clock dinner appointment that evening.

(It was already late Saturday afternoon.) Soon I was wheeled speedily to the delivery room; the *Pitocin* had finally worked. Behind the delivery table an anesthetist hovered over my head, repeating "Do you want a little gas? How about a little gas?" If I hadn't wanted any painkillers up until now I certainly wouldn't want one when I could push out my baby and see him being born in a matter of minutes. But I didn't have time to explain. I just waved her away each time I heard her questions.

Now the doctor was listening to the fetal heartbeat. He looked concerned. "O$_2$!" he yelled at the anesthetist. She quickly clamped a mask over my face, and, as if by reflex, I struggled to take if off. The doctor, seeing my lack of cooperation, had to lean over until his face was nearly on top of mine. "It's oxygen," he said. "Breathe deep. It's for the baby." So I complied. Almost immediately the baby was born. The doctor barely stayed long enough to shake my husband's hand. He still had time to make his dinner date. The baby had been born at 6:23 P.M. And, for my part, I was happy I had not been like some other mothers, too groggy to "breathe deep . . . for the baby."

I had been taught that after the baby was born the hard work was over. But in this case the ordeal was just beginning. It started as soon as I let it be known that I wished to go home when the baby and I were pronounced healthy, in a few hours if possible. A hush fell over the few remaining personnel in the delivery room. "Why do you want to do that?" a nurse asked me incredulously. I explained that I had an older child at home, that my husband was taking a week's vacation from his job to do the work I normally did, that I had intentions of resting in bed with the new baby and not doing much else, that I felt hospitals were for sick people, and that if I or the baby were not sick I knew I would be much more relaxed and get better rest in my own home. After hearing my answer, another nurse said I would have to be checked out by the resident who admitted me, since my doctor had left. My baby was taken away, and my husband and I were returned to the labor room. Then the procession began. Men, women, doctors, nurses came in to see me. Some doctors had wide-eyed interns a step behind, shaking their heads yes or no, seconding whatever a doctor would advise me. They would all begin the same way. "Are you the one who wants to go home? Why do you want to do that?" Then I would explain my feelings. Whenever they objected I would reply,

"I would be happy to stay if you can give me a medical reason," or "If there's a medical reason, I'll stay." One nurse forgot her second question. "Are you the one who wants to go home?" she asked me. I sighed and shook my head yes. She just stared at me for several minutes and left.

Meanwhile I tried to have the resident who admitted me located, to check met out. I was told alternately that he was having supper or unable to be located. As the fourth hour of waiting began my husband left me to start a personal search. The resident finally came in. "I hear you want to go home," he said. "Why do you want to do that?" I explained and he examined. "I don't want you to go home," he said. "I won't sign you out."

"What's wrong with me?" I asked.

"Nothing. But it's after ten. We'll talk about it in the morning."

"But I have to have a medical reason," I reminded him.

He looked at me for a long time. "I'll get you one," he said.

He returned a short time later and introduced me to a pediatrician. "So you want to go home," the pediatrician began.

"Is my baby all right?" I asked. "I'll stay only if there's a medical reason."

"I'll give you two," the pediatrican said. "He was born more than twelve hours after your water broke. So we want to check for infection. And he was over nine pounds. So we want to check for diabetes."

I was taken aback. I asked how long it would take to know.

"We'd like to observe him for twelve hours after birth," he said.

So I had been given my medical reasons. I felt tired and it was getting late. I agreed to stay overnight. The doctors left me alone, an intern nodding his head in approval as they made their way out.

"Where were you?" I was greeted by my roommates as I entered my assigned room. "Your baby's been crying the whole time."

It was then that I began to suspect I had been kept up in the labor room longer than necessary. I recalled from my first hospital birth that even the drugged woman next to me in the recovery room was monitored for only two hours before she was wheeled to her assigned room.

I asked the nurses if I could have my baby. They refused, saying that it was past feeding time. I said I just wanted to hold him, he had been crying for so long. After I promised not to feed him, they brought him to me to hold. When they left, I fed him. He nursed hungrily for a long time and fell asleep contentedly at my breast.

The nursery was attached to our mothers' room, and during the night there was always at least one baby crying. It was very hard to sleep because I always thought it was mine. The nurse refused to tell me whose baby was crying and refused to bring mine for the two A.M. feeding. She said he had been with me till midnight. She said I needed my rest. When it became apparent to her that I was not getting rest, she agreed to bring him, commenting, "I don't know what you could feed him. There's nothing in there anyway." Again, my baby nursed hungrily until he fell asleep at my breast.

The baby was taken away, and this time I was able to doze off, until I was awakened suddenly to have my temperature taken. The nurse examined my perineum and exclaimed that I was very swollen. The babies were brought for the six A.M. feeding and taken away. A doctor examining my swelling said that it had apparently been caused by the speedy birth of the baby's head due to the *Pitocin*. Breakfast arrived and, with it, ice packs for the lips of my vagina. They were very difficult to attach and to keep in place. By the time they were finally secured, they melted and had to be replaced. I asked when I could receive word on my baby's health, as twelve hours had passed since the birth, but I was told the doctors would not make their rounds till after nine. So, now it was to be more than twelve additional hours that I would stay.

At nine o'clock the babies were wheeled in to stay in the mothers' rooms for the most part of the day, because this hospital had daytime "rooming-in." My baby was sleeping on his side. A white fluid kept dripping out of his mouth. The nurse told me it was mucus and insisted that it was not formula. I had never known mucus to be so white. The baby slept till one in the afternoon.

The other babies were awake and screaming with hunger. However, the mothers were not permitted to feed them because it was "bath time." I was told I did not have to bathe my baby since I was newly delivered and had to get my rest. But the other mothers received instruction on how to smear their babies' bodies with oil. Then, it seemed to me, the babies really needed a bath.

An obstetrician—not mine, who was not on duty Sunday—came to check the swelling. "I thought you were going home," he said not unkindly. I explained to him about checking for infection and diabetes. "Do you have diabetes?" he asked. "No," I said. "Well, I just checked." He smiled, winked, and left. So, it was me, not the baby, who was suspected of having diabetes when a large baby was born. But no test was being taken. I felt I had been lied to. Now I was becoming more and more angry. And what of the baby's supposed infection? I began periodic trips to the nurses' station down the hallway or asked any hosptial staff members who came into the room. At first I was told that the doctors hadn't made their rounds yet. Later I was told they had already examined the babies and that I had missed them. Now, no pediatrician could be found.

As the morning wore on, I realized my husband hadn't phoned yet to make arrangements for picking up me and the baby. I began to feel abandoned by him; certainly I was not receiving support from anyone at the hospital, and I longed for a reassuring word. There was no phone in my room. I found a pay phone in the hallway and called my husband. He had just called the nurses' station on my floor, but they had told him it would be impossible to get a message to me, that if he wanted to speak to me, he could come at three P.M. for visiting hours.

During the morning, more hospital staff members came in and out, asking questions, staring, and offering their advice on why I should stay in the hospital. The best reason most could offer was that in their experience the soonest anyone went home was three days. No one could give a medical reason why I as an individual or my baby as an individual needed hospitalization.

I also began searching for an obstetrician to sign me out. According to the nurses I asked, obstetricians also were hard to find. Finally the resident from the night before was sent to me. I was relieved to see a familiar face, someone who knew what I was about. "I'll sign you out because your doctor told you that you could go home early if there was no medical reason to stay," he said. "But I'm glad to hear that the pediatrics department is not as irresponsible as the obstetrics department in this hospital." When I asked him what he meant, he said, "Any doctor who would agree to sign a woman out of this floor in less than three days is acting medically irresponsible." He signed for my doctor and left.

Shortly after one P.M., I was finally granted an audience with a member of the pediatrics staff. He invited me into the hallway and spoke in a hushed tone. 'What do you want?" he asked.

"How is my baby today?"

"He's fine."

"Then I would appreciate your signing him out. I've already been signed out myself."

"Let me speak to you, young lady," this doctor, who was about my age, began. He told me stories of the diseases babies could get in the first few days of life. The worst story involved "a strange factor in the blood" and ended in blood transfusions or muscular dystrophy. Something clicked in my mind during this last fantastic story. "But you're talking about physiologic jaundice," I said. "That's common to about seventy-five percent of all babies." Didn't he think I would have my baby under a pediatrician's care when I returned home? Didn't he think I would seek medical attention if my baby's coloring was very yellow? He seemed suprised I knew about physiologic jaundice

"Will you sign him out?" I asked again.

"No."

"If I wait till tonight. Then he will have been here twenty-four hours."

"No."

"Is there any way? Let me speak to the head pediatrician."

"Let me tell you," he said. "There is no way anyone on the pediatrics staff of this hospital will sign your baby out in less than three days."

I had heard what I needed to know. If I expected to leave the hospital in less than three days, I would have to take upon myself the responsibility of signing out my baby.

I made my decision known. More people came in to try to change my mind. But not one could offer a medical reason for staying. I enlisted the help of the head nurse to bring me the proper form for signing out the baby. She seemed to have a lot of difficulty finding the form. She did try to be helpful in her way. She brought me two disposable suction tubes to take home with me. "In case the baby turns blue," she explained.

Shifts changed and afternoon visiting hours began. My husband arrived to take me home. We were all ready, except for the form. At last it was located—a final, not-so-subtle, stunning piece of harassment. It was a three-part form, on one side of a sheet of paper. One part was entitled: DISPOSAL OF DEAD INFANT. The middle part was entitled: PERMISSION FOR DISPOSAL OF AMPUTATED MEMBER. And one part read: RELEASE.

I was nearly overcome by guilt at signing this "death form." The question—Are you sure you're doing the right thing?—wracked my mind. But mothers, or maybe all people, are sometimes imbued with a force that cannot, and should not, be repressed. Is it instinct? I only know that at that moment something must have been born in me, a belief in the rightness of my gut feelings as a woman and the importance of following those feelings. I signed quickly and left.

At home I felt exhausted, a quiet, peaceful, contented exhaustion, the kind one should feel after giving birth but that was only slowly coming over me now. That night I slept soundly, my baby beside me.

The next night I told my friend the story. Details like not having to have the episiotomy and nursing on the delivery table seemed unimportant next to the frustration and humiliation I had experienced. A hospital is a hospital and what had happened to me was the product of the hospital mentality. *"Never again,"* I remember telling my friend, not entirely aware of the significance of the conclusion I had reached. "The next one I'm having at home."

The next two years were spent reading about and researching home births. Writing a magazine cover story on the topic gave me the opportunity to speak to scores of doctors, nurses, midwives, parents, and other family members who had been connected with home birth. I attended my first home birth and was ready to write my story. About a week after it was published, I became pregnant for the third time.

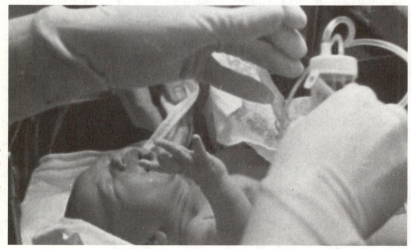

Suzanne Arms photograph

CHAPTER 2

"My Way"

I n the third month of my third pregnancy I went back to the
doctor who had delivered my second child. I took a chance
and asked him if he would deliver the baby at home. He did
not act surprised but said he was involved in a group practice and
could not commit himself to spending eight or nine hours at my
home. Besides, he said, his malpractice insurance did not cover the
home. But he was not against home deliveries, he added; in fact,
he looked at my medical records and said he was sure I would have
no trouble. But, no, there was no doctor he could recommend.

I saw this doctor one more time for a checkup, while I was still
seeking a birth attendant. For the two office visits the doctor
charged me one-fifth of his full fee for labor and delivery!

During two months of searching I spoke to many more people
connected with home birth. Some had delivered their own babies.
Others had had doctors who were no longer doing home deliveries.
Of those doctors still doing home birth, some were not taking on
new patients. Of those who would, the fees were exorbitant. Al-

though there sometimes seemed to be a number of possibilities open to me, doors closed quickly upon further investigation.

On four different occasions, I heard the name of the same doctor-and-nurse-midwife team or the health center with which they were connected. I was hesitant to follow through on these leads because I wasn't sure what I thought of a midwife-attended birth. I had to face it; I was prejudiced. I felt that a midwife wasn't as good as a doctor. Then a friend, a nurse, was examined by a midwife for a routine gynecological checkup. "It's a whole different world, " my friend said. "I would trust a midwife over any doctor I've had."

I was already in my sixth month when I called the midwife. She invited my husband and me to her apartment to discuss her services and our expectations. This *was* a whole different world. I had not yet encountered a doctor who would list his home phone number in a telephone directory. Certainly none had ever invited me to his home to discuss an upcoming birth.

Leaving Jane Davis's house, borrowed books under my arm, I felt a great relief. A home birth was now something real, something that was going to happen to me. We liked Jane; she had an appealing combination of professionalism and personal concern. She took her work seriously at the same time as she was friendly. She answered all our questions, including ones I wouldn't have dared ask a doctor. I asked about her schooling and her work experience (over 1,000 hospital deliveries and over two years of occasional home births) and requested phone numbers of women whose births she had attended. Then she asked us questions about how we regarded a home birth. Did my husband want to catch the baby? Did we want the older children to participate? "A home delivery is what you make it," Jane said. "I'm there to see that it's safe." I don't know why it surprised me that she asked no questions about my hospital experiences. I guess the reasons why one would want a home birth were just something understood.

After our initial visit I made an appointment for the required intake and examination by her supervising doctor at the health center. The baby and I were doing well, and I was given the medical go-ahead. I was examined at the center two more times toward the end of the pregnancy, once by a doctor and once by Jane. And on the night I was in labor Jane called the doctor when she arrived at my house, to put him on-call in case he had to meet me at the hospital.

Our other visits were to Jane's home. One of her chief concerns was nutrition. This was the first pregnancy in which someone asked me what I ate instead of caring only whether it kept my weight gain low. I had never stuck to the arbitrary diet sheets the doctors handed out. But I knew women who had subsisted on coffee and cigarettes for days before their monthly weigh-in, just so they wouldn't be "yelled at" by the doctor. One New York obstetrician, in fact, stamped pigs on the charts of women each month they gained more than two pounds. "Three pigs in a row," he threatened, "and I'll drop you as a patient."

Once under the midwife's care I was never even weighed. Instead, she asked me to write down everything I ate for a week. Then she reviewed my diet, adding up the number of grams of protein in the food I ate each day (I met her requirement of approximately 100 grams) and making suggestions where my intake of a particular vitamin seemed minimal. She never acted dogmatic or judgmental. Having met my share of Adelle Davis fans and vegetarians, I was fearful Jane would criticize my occasional indulgence in cake or processed food. Instead, she stuck to the information I gave her, and from what I appeared to like she recommended increased amounts of certain foods, such as green leafy vegetables to raise the amount of iron I ingested, or nuts and peanut butter for vitamin B.

About six weeks before my due date we moved to a new apartment. Now I could picture the birth, where the bassinet would be, who would sit where. It seemed believable that it would be real, that "two months from now in this very bed a baby of mine will have been born. . . ."

But what of this baby born on this bed? Was it fair to deny him—just in case—all the expensive hospital machinery, for partly selfish reasons? Early in my pregnancy, a man I had met only once asked me directly if I thought what I planned to do was safe. I fumbled with a positive answer, trying to come up with something convincing. In my mind I became defensive, and I felt angry at him for causing me to deal with the realities of guilt and death. I thought, "Who is he to try to deny my years of knowledge, experience, and conviction?" I decided to have an answer prepared. To anyone who dared throw me off-guard again, I would say, "Do you think I would risk the life of my baby, and my life, if I thought this wasn't safe?"

Surprisingly, no one else ever asked. But that didn't mean I didn't have to deal with the issue anyway, not only in my thoughts but also in late-night conversations with my husband and in dreams in which I would find myself in a strange hospital bed.

I was entirely convinced there was no need for the hospital as long as everything went well; I knew I could labor and give birth and recuperate and that my baby would get better care in the relaxed and secure atmosphere of our home. But that was if everything went normally. What of complications?

There were two types of complications, I decided: those caused by interference and those that originated with the mother, the baby, or the pregnancy. It was easy for me to dispense with those caused by interference with the normal process of labor and birth, things like unnecessary medications and delivery-table position— I had dispensed with them when I dispensed with the hospital procedure. Of those that were not caused by interference, most seemed either predictable or preventable. That was why I was following a healthy diet and that was why the doctor or the midwife listened to my heartbeat and the baby's or took my blood pressure.

What then of the rare complications that might not be preventable or predictable? What of premature separation of the placenta, causing hemorrhage for the mother and possible death to her and the baby? Well, folic acid, one study showed, had seemed to prevent the condition, and I was taking folic acid tablets. And a warning show of blood almost always preceded the big hemorrhage in this condition. And the doctor would be waiting to alert the hospital and meet me there if I needed a cesarean operation or a transfusion. However long it would take me to get to the hospital was not much longer than it would take to set up for an emergency operation, even if I were already in the hospital. My mind produced the answers almost before the questions had formed. What if the baby didn't breathe after birth? But I was not ingesting medication, so the breathing wouldn't be depressed. But what if it should be anyway, from some other cause? That was the reason the midwife would be there, in case something went wrong. Even a respected doctor had said that hospital resuscitators could do no better than trained human hands if a baby is not able eventually to start breathing on her own.

It helped that the statistics available were on my side. The number of infant deaths was higher in the hospital than in the home.

And the number of maternal deaths was also higher. Questions, answers, bouncing back and forth. Indeed, on reflection, it seemed as if home births might be *safer* than hospital births. Home births safer than hospital births? Yes, I could say it and believe it—the statistics, the medical studies, the interviews, the personal experience, all confirmed one another. Home birth, for the healthy mother who was determined to be heading for a normal birth and baby, appeared safer than hospital birth. I had come to believe it was so.

Noontime on a not-too-warm, not-too-cold Monday I pushed my two-year-old son in the stroller while my five-year-old walked beside me. At the school eight blocks away, I told his kindergarten teacher, "I think I might be in labor. So maybe someone else will pick him up at three." Constipation-type cramps—no sensation in the belly area—were characteristic of labor for me, and at my son's school it was still too soon to be sure of what I was feeling. Leaving the classroom, I turned back for one last word with the teacher: "By the way, if he comes to school tomorrow and is all excited about seeing the baby born, please do believe him. We're having the baby at home."

I returned home and telephoned my husband at his office. "I'm really not sure," I told him, "but if you're planning on eating lunch out. . . ." He said he would rather not take a chance; he would leave for home in time to pick up our kindergartener at school. While the younger son took an afternoon nap, I telephoned my husband's brother and his wife and asked them to come over at the end of their workday. They had agreed to care for the children during my labor, and my brother-in-law would take photographs if there was time for that, too. "Check with me before you leave work," I said. "I'm still not sure."

As the afternoon continued, I decided I wasn't the right type of person to have a home birth. After all, I hated to bother people, especially if I couldn't be sure it was necessary. It would be embarrassing to call the midwife and ask her to come all the way to my home only to discover I wasn't really in labor. But by four o'clock I decided to call. My husband and two boys were at home and watching me. The momentum of events of the day seemed to tell me I was indeed in labor. I called Jane's answering service, they beeped her, and she called me from a store. She would finish looking over some fabric and take the subway to my home. Jane arrived at around six, along with my brother-in-law and sister-in-law. The cast of characters had assembled. It looked like the drama was about to begin.

The midwife examined me on my bed and announced that I was four (out of ten) centimeters dilated. However, the baby's head was high, and my contractions, though three minutes apart, were not strong. My husband made dinner. The midwife said I could eat it, but what I really felt like having was an apple and a cup of hot tea.

After dinner and cleanup and a bath from Daddy, the children retired to their bedroom for quiet games with their aunt and uncle. The midwife, my husband, and I timed my contractions on the living room couch. Everyone moved around the apartment at will, including the children. The atmosphere was serene and pleasant.

When the contractions became more intense, at about nine, I changed to my "birth outfit," a loose-fitting long wraparound robe, and my husband prepared our bed. We three shifted to our sleeping alcove off the living room. My husband and I stayed on the bed, me crouched over some pillows, panting through contractions, his fists pressed on my lower back to help alleviate my third "back labor." Jane faced us in a chair, alternately listening to the baby's heart with her fetoscope, making a suggestion or two for my comfort, sipping coffee, or dozing. The two boys wandered in and out, the five-year-old demonstrating an empathy we will always remember, whispering, stroking my face and legs, smiling in approval at the end of a contraction. The younger boy observed for moments in silence, then returned to play. Only once do I recall commenting, "Please don't let him crash into me," feeling nervous that he might take a running leap onto the bed, as two-year-olds sometimes do—but this time during a contraction.

As midnight approached I began to feel nausea and the sensation of having to move my bowels—both signs I was in transition, a name for the end of the first part of labor. After several more contractions the midwife examined me and told me I could begin to push, slowly and gently. But I was anxious to see the baby by this time, and I was not used to controlling my pushing. I listened to her and sometimes pushed gently; at other times I pushed harder than I ever had in my life, feeling bad for not obeying her. Other times I did a breathing pattern through a contraction as a way of trying not to push at all. This was a kind of labor I hadn't planned for—a slow labor. Having my third baby, relaxed and in my own home, I had expected ease and speed. This was new, a slow birth. And I was unaccustomed to taking directions from Jane. "I'm trying hard to do what you say," I told her. My sister-in-law later told me her memory of the birth was how slowly the head was born. This was one area of the midwife's expertise I didn't appreciate until daybreak when, after urinating for the first time since the baby's birth, I was able to wipe myself with toilet paper, not a squeeze bottle of water, as after my hospital births. At home the slow birth directed by the midwife had allowed my skin to stretch gradually without becoming painfully sore.

As the expulsion stage of my labor grew longer, I began to feel anxious and impatient. Jane checked the baby's heartbeat periodically, and I almost expected to hear her say that something was not normal, but she always assured me everything was well. The head was harder than most newborns' heads, she could feel and see that, she said. So it took a little longer to be born. And the head was probably rotating itself first; it had been in a posterior position and that was why I had experienced back labor. So, I kept repeating to myself; the head was high, it was slower to come down . . . hard, rotating, and slow. I knew these explanations made sense. But I began to curse anyway. "Where is this baby already?" Jane and my husband both assured me they could see the head with each contraction, but I only half believed them. I knew that, contrary to the midwife's orders, some of my pushes were bulldozer pushes, all-encompassing thrusts that seemed to start from my toes and bowels and brain, all ending at that one hard, rotating, slow head. *So, why was it taking so long?*

My second stage of labor, the expulsion stage, lasted forty minutes. The pushing stages for my two other babies had been about fifteen minutes each. It was thus with relief, not pure ecstasy, that my third baby was guided into the world. Finally, I had felt the longed-for burning sensation. I gave harder pushes for the hard head. Finally, I felt my midwife and my husband each take one of my feet and push my knees toward my shoulders, altering the angle of my sitting position. "Ah, this is how she has to push," I heard Jane say. More burning, another contraction, more burning. Then, finally, the most burning of all, my skin and muscles seeming to burst apart, the bottom splitting open to let a head be born, then a body slip out. I heard "ooohs" and "ahhs." One part of my mind told the other, "You have to open your eyes to see your baby." So my eyes opened. There was a still bundle of greasy flesh, limbs pasted around a rectangular trunk. A midwife with a bulb syringe was drawing mucus out of a new baby's nose and mouth, nose again, mouth again. It was my baby. It didn't move. But it would, when it started to breathe the air. I knew it would be soon. Now the face was moving. It was starting. Everyone was silent.

What was it? I couldn't see; was it a boy or a girl? The midwife waved aside my question with her hand. Was cleaning mucus more important than knowing the sex of my child? Now the midwife was done, and she looked down at the lively form: "It's a boy." More "oohs" and "ahhs." Well, I had heard those words before. But this time the baby was still mine, it was still my boy, still attached to my insides and now being handed to me. I slid him up my belly till his mouth found my nipple, and we were a full circle, the breast, the baby, the umbilical cord, placenta, all attached.

Then the placenta separated and came out; the circle was broken. And then the cord, it had stopped throbbing, it had to go, too; it was useless. Two clamps were fastened and in between them my husband cut the dead cord. So even less of the circle remained. The baby let go of my breast and so even less. Though my arms held him, he seemed to lie there alone against my body. Slowly he had become alive, become a life of his own.

He was passed to his father, another full circle. Reality set in: *what if I bleed?* I was sitting in wetness. "You lost about a pint and a half of blood, about a half a pint more than normal." The midwife gave me a shot of *Pitocin* in my thigh to supplement the natural contractions and help prevent any further unnecessary bleeding. (Before she left three hours later I took a tablet of *Ergotrate* to help contract my uterus also, and I took another one at eight in the morning.) *But what if I still hemorrhaged?* Jane showed me I could massage my uterus to a hard ball. I was breastfeeding and that would also contract my uterus. I knew all this by rote, and yet I was scared. Scared of going to that hospital, any hospital. "I guess this is the last thing left that could go wrong, and that's why I'm afraid," I said.

The new baby was returned to me. We all toasted with champagne to the new little life, 9 lb. 12 oz. of life. A two-year-old boy, now known as my middle son, watched me. "Come up on the bed,"

I invited him with a nonbreastfeeding arm. "It's wet," he said. But he could be coaxed on. My oldest boy didn't wait for an invitation. He came up to sit close to me, his head on my shoulder, a hand on his smallest brother (still naked, never even washed off), and rested with us.

Then all those other people were hungry, and they wanted to eat. I didn't. Jane insisted I have at least some warm milk, and holding up my head, she fed it to me. But I preferred to lie back in the wet, occasionally moving my baby from breast to breast. I was exhausted, and what I wanted to do most was bask in the coziness of life and wetness and the good sense of doing something I really believed in. People came and went from my bed, joked, kissed, changed my clothes. By the time they were ready to leave I was feeling stronger, after the most exhausting pushing I had done in my life. I wanted to sit up and talk about it now, but it was 4 A.M., and they were exhausted, too, and left for their homes. So I lay down again, the baby on one side of me, and on the other, my man, in a thick, hard sleep.

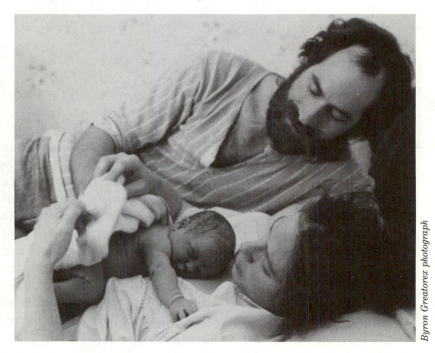

Byron Greatorex photograph

CHAPTER 3

A Historical
Perspective

E ven before the Egyptians began keeping records we can
guess that women simply helped other women give birth
at home. In fact, this is the situation in most places in the
world today. What recorded history does show us is the slow evolution of birth in this country from a woman-dominated, family
experience in the home, which was not usually very safe or pleasant
should a serious complication of labor or delivery present itself, to
a male-dominated, medical experience in the hospital which is not
usually very safe or pleasant if a serious complication of labor and
delivery does not present itself. The problem, then, has become
one of balance: if the male-dominated medical establishment, after
remarkable and necessary developments and discoveries such as
hospitals and anesthesia, had saved these advances for true complications of birth, the current home birth movement might never
have had to begin. It was at the beginning of this century when
the balance began to be disturbed—when the doctors began to eat

away at the normal childbearing population, drawing it under the umbrella of sickness, medicine, and hospitalization. It was the beginning of an era when, as one prominent pediatrician has put it, many doctors felt "pregnant women should be treated for their fetus as if it were an abnormal growth causing undesirable symptoms."[1]

It is not that home birth proponents are against advances in medicine. From the first successful cesarean operation performed at home by a man on his wife in 1500 A.D. to the cesareans occurring right now in sterile hospital operating rooms, millions of mothers and their children can point to the developments of modern medicine for rescuing them in a life-threatening situation. But home birth proponents are against *misusing* the advances of medicine. Too often nowadays when we visit a new mother in the hospital, trying to recuperate from her C-section scars as fast as her postoperative neighbor in the next bed, she explains matter-of-factly, "I was in labor for eleven hours." What used to be considered within the range of *normal* labor time is now justification for major surgery with all its inherent risks.

The question is: What is normal? Newborn babies with bluish toes and fingers are considered normal. A mother's feeling of depression after birth, commonly called "postpartum blues," is normal. A 30 percent cesarean rate at a city's major teaching hospital is now considered normal. Have American women's bodies changed so much that one in three or four of us is now incapable of giving birth vaginally? The answer is that medicine has come so far from what is normal in childbirth that most doctors have probably never seen a natural, normal birth. Most doctors have never seen a birth at home. They need to learn that there is a place for home birth and a place for hospital birth. And the place for home birth is with at least 90 percent of childbearing women.

That was about the percentage who gave birth at home at the turn of the century. Already by that time half of all births were being attended by doctors. Many midwives had been purged as witches over the previous 150 years. Doctors helped to propagate the myth that midwives were, at best, ignorant old nannies or, at worst, ignorant unclean evildoers. We see an extension of such attitudes today among doctors who belittle a woman's opinions of childbirth if she is "just a mother."

What the doctor's view of history often neglects to mention is that doctors were the ones responsible for the tens of thousands of deaths due to childbed (puerperal) fever in the nineteenth century and even into the twentieth. Ignacz Semmelweis had to discover that this widespread killer disease was caused by improper, unsanitary scrubbing procedures as doctors went from examining cadavers to examining laboring women. But the conservative medical profession viewed suspiciously the discovery of antisepsis, and it would be many years before puerperal fever was virtually eliminated. Doctors were reluctant to institute a sensible change that could have saved countless lives.

Besides the discrediting of midwives, advances in medical technology, such as the discovery of anesthesia, made it easier for doctors to convince their patients that they were the superior birth attendants and the hospital the superior birth place. Some doctors truly felt that it was a better place for giving birth, in case medical intervention was needed. But others were motivated by less noble reasons: obstetrics and gynecology, particularly in surgery, were fast becoming lucrative fields. And even a general practitioner could see that a doctor's time could be spent more efficiently if a woman gave birth in the hospital. He could attend to several medical tasks and receive assistance from nurses and orderlies for the "dirty work" during the same time it would take to sit at one woman's bedside for a home birth.

Since that time, there have always been women who would not think of having their babies at the hospital in any case and those who couldn't afford the hospital. But, for the most part, middle- and upper-income mothers began preferring the hospital to the home for the business of birthing. Hospital birth became a matter of status. The ideal picture was of the newly delivered mother awakening from a painless labor and birth and pampered at bedside for one to two weeks, with only an occasional meeting with that drippy, messy new baby. Never mind if drugs were dangerous for the mother or baby, if constant bed rest for the mother was bad for her circulation and could cause hemorrhage, or if bonding between the mother and baby could be forfeited by the lack of early contact. Hospital birth was propagandized by doctors as intelligent, luxurious, and liberating. And it was—for them. The statistical portrait of birth in America reflected the gradual change: by the time the first fifty years of the century had passed, well over half of all births were attended by doctors, in hospitals. During this time the infant and maternal mortality rate dropped, and the medical establishment was quick to take the credit. But it is more likely that the establishment of prenatal care and blood banks, a generally improved diet, and the discovery of antibiotics led to a healthier child-bearing population.

Again, what the doctor's view of the history of birth does not mention is that while hospital mortality and morbidity were being lowered, the rate of deaths at home was lower still. During the first half of the century several home birth services were in operation, chiefly for those women too poor or too far away to have their babies in hospitals. Two of the best known were the Chicago Maternity Center, serving inner-city women, and the Frontier Nursing Serice in Kentucky, serving Appalachian women. It is not easy for the medical establishment to explain how, in our increasingly wealthy and highly technical society, these low-key home birth services could boast lower maternal and infant mortality statistics than the hospitals. But they did. A 1932 report prepared by the Metropolitan Life Insurance Company on 10,000 births covered by the Frontier Nursing Service, for example, showed an infant death rate of 9.1 per 10,000 live births, while both the national average and the Kentucky state-wide average during the same period was 34 per 10,000 live births.[2] At the Chicago Maternity Center over 12,000 births were attended between 1950 and 1960, without one maternal mortality. At that time the national average was two per 1,000. Another well-known comparison of the relative safety of home birth was published in 1933 by the New York Academy of Medicine.[3] The total maternal mortality rate, the maternal mortality from infection, and the rate of mortality due to hemorrhage were all significantly lower at home. It is important to note that almost all the mothers in these home birth services were from poor homes, usually approaching confinement with several high-risk conditions.

Today, the most recent figures available from the "Annual Summary of Vital Statistics" that appears in the journal, *Pediatrics,* show that the United States, where more than 90 percent of all births now take place in a hospital, is seventeenth in the world in infant mortality.[4] The top three spots on the same table, indicating lowest infant mortality, were claimed by Japan, Sweden, and Finland, countries where the professional midwife plays an active role in maternity care and in promoting breastfeeding.

THE "NATURAL" CHILDBIRTH MOVEMENT

Anyone looking at such statistics can see that there is a crying need for change in the American way of birth. Early ripples for change were stirred by the writings of the British doctor, Grantly Dick-Read. He argued that pain in childbirth was caused by lack of knowledge, leading to fear, leading to tension, leading finally to pain. He suggested education for the birthing mother which would reduce her fear, causing less tension and less pain. This would reduce the need for drugs and eliminate their inherent risks to mother and baby. But the few women in the United States who were exposed to Dick-Read's ideas were usually dismissed in the typical fashion by their doctors. As late as 1960, one doctor writing a book on obstetrics history referred to a "fad of hypnotism" or "mesmerism" in childbirth around the time chloroform, an early anesthetic, was introduced. "Today there is a revival of 'mesmerism' in a sense, by such methods as those of Dick-Read . . ." the doctor wrote, in his only reference to childbirth preparation for the mother in his book.[5]

Also across the ocean, but a number of years later than Dick-Read's discoveries, a French doctor named Fernand Lamaze observed a set of exercises used by laboring women in Russia. Lamaze introduced the Pavlov method to France in 1951, and it was introduced into this country in 1959 by Marjorie Karmel in her engaging book, *Thank You, Dr. Lamaze*. But in the passive fifties, not many women were ready for active participation in an event so earthy as childbirth. It just seemed easier to have faith in doctors and technology and revel in the prosperity of the status quo.

The exceptions, again, were those few women whose feelings told them home birth was better and poor women or women who lived great distances from hospitals, who were of necessity continuing to have their babies at home. But it was always assumed by the establishment that, given the choice, these poor women would rather have had a hospital delivery with a doctor, which in some cases was true.

THE HOME BIRTH MOVEMENT

One small-town girl whose name is now Lee Stewart was growing up in Missouri at the time. Her birth place had been her parents' bed in an old farmhouse in Lutesville, a town which still has a population of only 600. With memories of the births of her siblings who followed her, Lee Stewart and her husband David chose unattended home birth each time when their own five children were born, because they could not find a hospital to meet their needs or a physician or midwife to come to their home. When the Stewarts moved East during their childbearing years, there followed a steady stream of letters from people requesting information, encouragement, and support. Sensing a growing tide, the Stewarts began the International Association of Parents and Professionals for Safe Alternatives in Childbirth (NAPSAC). In 1976, more than 500 people from twenty-eight states and Canada and Australia gathered across the Potomac from Washington, D.C. for the first NAPSAC conference to hear midwives, doctors, and parents support alternatives to hospital birth such as maternity homes. But the most support went to home birth. The NAPSAC meeting marked the first time organized, nationwide support was given to the growing home birth movement. NAPSAC held a tenth-anniversary conference in Chicago in 1986 and to this day remains the largest international organization whose main purpose is to act as a clearinghouse for alternative birth information. Back in Missouri, the Stewarts now devote full time to answering mail, reviewing literature, and writing articles and to related issues like home schooling.

Besides the birth of the Stewarts' first child, the sixties also saw the birth of movements for social change. College students graduating from campus reform movements then went on to form the core of other movements. The increasing desire of women to control their own bodies, of patients to have a say in what is done to them by doctors, and of all people to understand more fully the quality of their lives have also pointed to the home birth movement.

Women's and patients' rights and the back-to-nature movements have set the atmosphere for home birth, but the most significant catalyst was the gradual acceptance of childbirth preparation in hospitals. Whether consciously or not, once women saw that they could cause radical changes in birth practices in a relatively short period of time, simply by demanding them, a revival of birth in the home was a logical extension.

Acceptance of the Lamaze method began in 1960 when author Marjorie Karmel, along with Elisabeth Bing, probably the best-known Lamaze teacher in the country, formed the American Society for Psychoprophylaxis in Obstetrics (ASPO). ASPO-certified teachers went out into the community to disseminate "the Lamaze method" through instruction in the physiology of birth and a series of complex breathing patterns. By 1970 the missionary zeal of Lamaze converts was filling classes in many areas of the country. And in the western United States, excited parents flocked to the office of Dr. Robert Bradley of Denver, whose own "Bradley method" pioneered the idea of the child's father as the mother's most important "coach," right into the delivery room.

Most obstetricians at first resisted "prepared childbirth," as it is usually called, in every way they knew how. Writing in a hospital magazine on the subject of fathers in the delivery room, one physician stated flatly that a delivery room is an operating room and that unnecessary personnel increased the chance of infection, interfered with his teaching of residents and interns, and increased his chances of being sued. He questioned whether the motive of a man wanting to be with his wife for the birth of their child was "sightseeing." Across the United States some fathers sued in court for the right to be with their wives in the delivery room, but the courts said that each hospital had the right to make its own decision in the matter. In California John Quinn handcuffed himself to his wife and hid the key when it was time for her to be brought to the delivery room. In 1973 in the United States Congress, Rep. Martha Griffiths (D., Mich.) introduced a bill providing that any hospital receiving federal funds must allow the biological father to attend the birth of his child if the mother consents. There are still hospitals where this is not guaranteed, and there are even some which forbid an unmarried mother to bring a friend or sister with her. Still, in virtually every major area of the country, in both large cities and small towns, there now are doctors and hospitals who will allow their patients to practice prepared childbirth. While this still leaves the option under physician control, and while too often a mother's intentions are sabotaged by the hospital or her doctor's interference, on the whole the idea of being conscious for delivery is once again acceptable, due almost entirely to consumer pressure.

As the student movement of the sixties was treated in flamboyant California style by much media attention, so too did the media spotlight California birth events as news. Californian Norman Casserley, a male midwife, had been delivering babies for about twenty-five years, but it wasn't until his 1971 arrest for practicing medicine without a license and his later conviction and appeal that the media attention for himself translated into publicity for the home birth cause. The same year of Casserley's arrest saw a group of midwives practicing in the Santa Cruz area join together to form the Birth Center, where prenatal care, labor, delivery at home attended by an experienced midwife or two, and family-planning and new-parent discussion groups were available for thirty-five dollars. Following the successful publication of *Birth Book* by Birth Center midwife Raven Lang, California undercover agents arrested three Birth Center midwives and raided the office, creating more sympathy and publicity for the issue.[6] Spiritually but not physically close to the Birth Center was another self-taught California midwife, Nancy Mills, who, after hundreds of births, won the respect of her community and a national reputation. One television network evening news program featured a segment on a Nancy Mills-attended home birth. And, finally, Californian Suzanne Arms wrote *Immaculate Deception*. Still in print and making waves in consumer and medical circles, the book is a seething indictment of the American way of birth.

From the East Coast, booklets like *The Cultural Warping of Childbirth* by Doris Haire, a co-founder of the International Childbirth Education Association, and early articles by sociologist Barbara Katz Rothman added fuel to the fire. Parent support groups like Home Oriented Maternity Experience and the Association for Childbirth at Home began to spring up, with chapters dotting the country. The middle classes had begun to become aware of the benefits of home birth. Anthropologist Lester Hazell, in her published demographic study of a home birth population in California, found that 90 percent lived in single-family houses where the father worked outside the home and the families owned one or two cars and were not on welfare.[7] The idea of home birth had entered American mainstream thinking.

Today, it is no longer unheard of to see favorable articles on home birth, both in the popular press and the medical literature. Beginning with Jack Anderson's Christmas Eve 1978 column entitled "No Hospital Birth? How Dare Joseph and Mary!" the popular press has had good things to say about home birth, including stories on water births and celebrities who have had babies at home. As the baby boomers of the '50s reach childbearing age, a glut of books on childbirth is flooding the market, including several just on home birth. Most of the many general childbirth books at least mention home birth as a viable option, and books like *A Good Birth, A Safe Birth,* by Diana Korte and Roberta Scaer, routinely advise against interventions and advocate the protection of a written parents' birth plan.[8] In the groves of academe, the City University of New York awarded a Ph.D. to Keri Lipkowitz in 1986 for her thesis, "Interpretation and Critique of the Choice and Experience of Home Birth: Positive Home Birth Experiences of New York Women."

The turnabout in the medical literature has been even more dramatic. In the '70s, when physician Lewis Mehl conducted an investigation into more than 1,000 matched samples of women having home and hospital births, he spent years trying to get a well-known medical journal to publish it. But the '80s have seen the publication of several reports showing the safety of home birth—"Home Delivery and Neonatal Mortality in North Carolina" and "Neontal Outcome in Planned *vs.* Unplanned Out-of-Hospital Births in Kentucky," both of which appeared in the *Journal of the AMA,* and "Four Years Experience with Home Birth by Licensed Midwives in Arizona," which appeared in the *Journal of the American Public Health Association.*[9]

Unfortunately, reality is still far behind the published literature, and many physicians will not even give prenatal care to a mother planning a home birth or meet her at the hospital in an emergency. If these doctors truly cared about the safety and health of mothers and babies, wouldn't they want these women to receive their services? As recently as ten years ago, most obstetricians simply said that a home birth movement didn't exist or wasn't growing, or if it did and was, there was no need to take it seriously. One is reminded of the medical establishment's reactions for so many years to abortion and birth control; it denied that a need existed.

Some doctors who care enough to resist tried to reform the hospitals. Reacting to a growing number of home birth families he had met, obstetrician Richard Aubry, working through the American College of Obstetricians and Gynecologists, was influential in encouraging hospitals to create "birthing rooms," which are informally furnished, unlike delivery rooms, which are really operating rooms. Aubry's plan was also to allow young children to visit their mothers and newborn siblings in the hospital. Many hospitals reacted well to these ideas, hoping to lure home birth-inclined couples back to hospital birth. Although instituting these procedures, and in some cases allowing certified nurse-midwives to gain privileges at a hospital, have benefitted some families choosing hospital birth, in some communities they are like window dressing, and the birthing room is rarely used or the midwife is allowed to deliver only on Fridays.

But the latest and most organized reaction to the growing home birth movement has been to fight and to try to kill it. Obstetricians' reliance on technology and the manyfold increase in both cesarean operations and medical malpractice insurance rates have combined to make any threat to universal, doctor-controlled hospital birth a threat on an economic level.

The first sign of an aggressive, organized reaction on the part of the medical community came with the release of a flimsy report from the American College of Obstetricians and Gynecologists purportedly showing a two-to-five times greater risk with home rather than hospital delivery. Widely publicized as a "study," it was actually a press release reporting statistics from selected states where "out-of-hospital" births might include late miscarriages or births in taxis but very few planned home births among healthy couples with trained midwives, as later scientific research would report in medical journals. But the "ACOG study" did receive wide publicity because the press release was on the stationery of a respected medical organization.[10] Also receiving publicity was a comment by ACOG president Warren Pearse that home birth is "child abuse." This climate led to the abduction of a home-born baby by child welfare authorities in Houston in 1982.

When tactics such as these didn't stem the growing home birth movement, organized medicine went even further. If a home-born baby died, even when the parents did not blame the practitioner and even when there was nothing more a doctor in a hospital could have done to save the baby, murder charges would be brought against the midwife or doctor through the district attorney's office, acting under the influence of the medical lobby. This happened across the land: to a physician in Alaska, to midwives in Florida and California, and to three midwives in Canada, among others. Although there might be a conviction on a lesser charge, such as practicing medicine without a license for a lay midwife, or complete dismissal of charges, the time and money spent in defense and the emotional and physical drain to the practitioner could be insurmountable, and the medical establishment would be successful in squelching that practice. This is in sharp contrast to the death of a newborn occurring in a hospital, where routine questions at a weekly meeting would suffice, and the obstetrician would continue in practice—business as usual. Not as dramatic as murder charges, in other cases doctors helping at home births might find their hospital privileges revoked or their licenses suspended, with equally great toll on finances, health, and livelihood. Although there might be a groundswell of popular support for the home birth physician, such as New York's family practitioner George Wootan, whose story appeared on "60 Minutes," there might not be enough influence or money to mount an adequate defense. A founding doctor of the short-lived Alternative Birth Crisis Coalition commented, "We are like a small-town fire department dousing a small blaze here and there when meanwhile the ACOG is starting a forest fire across the country." In truth, organized medicine has top-flight, paid lobbyists representing it at every major legislature in the country, including the federal government, while the supporters of alternative medicine are mostly parents with babes in arms donating money from the food budget for a defense fund. Groups like the Health Alternatives Legal Foundation hope to offset some of the financial burden to individual practitioners by sponsoring some defenses.

As this decade ends, home birth advocates draw sustenance from their ability to survive in such a climate of persecution. They look forward to and participate in events like the First International Conference on Homebirth in London in October 1987. It appears that as long as women give birth, they will want to choose where, with whom, and how they do it.

CHAPTER 4

A Look at the Hospitals

Sheila Willis, also known as Patient No. 34688527, arrived at the University Medical Center with her husband, Tim, at 2:10 A.M. Actually, she was dropped off at the front door since he had to find a parking space for their car. This wasn't always easy in the big city, even at night. It was no telling how far she'd have had to walk from the parking spot, and walking did not appeal to her now that she was in active labor.

It was their first baby, and Sheila knew she would probably not have a fast birth, so they had stayed home for early labor, as the Lamaze teacher had suggested. Labor had begun eight hours earlier, with the sudden warm gush of the bag of waters as Sheila had been preparing dinner. Tim had eaten both their portions since Sheila had been warned not to eat anything during labor in case she needed general anesthesia. Now contractions were about five minutes apart and Sheila's doctor had told her over the phone that it was time she headed down to the hospital for a "look-see." Sheila's heart had pounded excitedly when she left for the hospital. It

31

seemed hard for her to believe the baby was really going to be born this day.

Sheila felt afraid, waiting on the barren sidewalk, so she entered the hospital's main lobby. Having entered, she had a contraction and began panting as she had been taught in Lamaze class. "Can I help you?" asked the woman at the reception desk. When the contraction had passed, Sheila said, "No, thank you. I'm waiting for my husband." The woman smiled and said, "No time for that. Come here and give me your name."

Sheila went over to the desk, sat down, and gave the woman her name. The woman found her file and began asking Sheila questions which hadn't already been answered on the form, such as if and when Sheila's amniotic membranes, which Sheila knew meant bag of waters, had broken. Twice as Sheila answered she'd had to lean over at an angle and grip the table edge as a contraction took hold of her. She wished Tim would arrive. A wheelchair came, and Sheila sat in it. "Thank you," said the orderly. "The last lady tried to refuse my ride. We had some time convincing her that no lady comes on the maternity floor without a wheelchair. We can't take that responsibility."

He wheeled Sheila into an elevator and then upstairs to an examining room on the maternity floor and left. A nurse greeted Sheila by name, helped her from the chair to the examining table, and placed her feet in the stirrups. Two men dressed in surgical greens came in. One nodded a greeting and held out his hand, which the nurse covered with a sterile glove. He inserted it into Sheila and spoke quietly to the other man. Then he pulled out his hand and let the nurse take off the glove. Sheila had another contraction and began panting and blowing. She remained in the same position on the table while the resident, as he must have been, made a phone call from the corner of the room. "I have your Mrs. Willis here," he began. Sheila heard words like "start the Pit." The doctor hung up and turned around to the nurse. "Take Mrs. Willis to the labor room," he said, giving Sheila's leg a couple of friendly slaps. "She ruptured a long time ago. I'll give instructions for the IV."

The doctor left and the nurse took Sheila's feet out of the stirrups. "Is my doctor here?" Sheila asked. "That was he on the phone," said the nurse. She helped Sheila back into the wheelchair and wheeled her to another room that looked like the first but a little smaller. Sheila was relieved to find Tim already waiting there. She immediately had a contraction, but this time she just panted. Tim stared at her with a worried and loving look.

Sheila was helped out of the wheelchair and asked to undress and place her clothes and personal belongings in a brown bag. She was given a short hospital gown to put on and directed to the bathroom. Sheila changed in there and came out holding the back of the hospital gown to make the two sides meet. The nurse helped Sheila up onto the bed and pulled up its side. Sheila felt like an overgrown baby in a crib. The nurse left, and Tim came over and held Sheila's hand.

Another nurse came in, and Tim backed off. The new nurse said, "Time for your miniprep." She pulled down the side rail, separated Sheila's knees, placed her feet flat on the sheets and pushed them back toward her thighs. Sheila had to fall back on her elbows to catch her balance. The nurse began shaving Sheila's pubic hair. Sheila was glad it didn't take long and that she didn't have a contraction because she was afraid she would move while the razor was there. When the nurse finished she left, and Tim came over and helped Sheila back to a sitting position.

Then the nurse returned, and Tim moved away again. "Here is your enema," said the nurse. She administered it to Sheila and then quickly helped her off the bed. The hospital gown was falling off the front of Sheila's shoulders, but the nurse was rushing Sheila toward the bathroom again. "Now I want you to sit there a full twenty minutes," she told Sheila. "I don't want you out one minute sooner. I want you all emptied out. Don't forget now." The nurse closed the bathroom door. Tim asked Sheila if she'd mind if he got something to eat so he wouldn't feel dizzy later and she agreed.

Sitting on the toilet, Sheila tried to lift her feet onto the edge of the seat because she felt uncomfortable with them on the floor. They seemed too low down. During her first ten minutes on the toilet she'd had two contractions. Each time she blew out she heard water spurting into the toilet. She wasn't sure if it was coming from her vagina or her anus. After the second contraction she began to wonder how long twenty minutes would be. She had put her watch in the brown bag. She decided to count to sixty ten times and then leave the bathroom. She counted through two more contractions, panting as they came. She enjoyed counting and panting in rhythm and was glad the enema wasn't as bad as someone in the Lamaze class had made it out to be. After the second contraction Sheila left the bathroom in a happier frame of mind and climbed back into the bed. She decided she would count and pant in rhythm for all the contractions she would have until Tim came back.

But thinking of Tim eating produced a strong wave of nausea in her. When a contraction began, she didn't start to pant because she was afraid it would cause her to vomit. Instead she grabbed the bars of the bed and sucked in little breaths of air, a sort of reverse panting, which she thought would prevent her from vomiting. When the contraction ended and her eyes cleared, she realized the nurse was at the door looking at her. "I'm nauseous," Sheila said, louder than she thought it would sound. The nurse smiled and said, "It's too soon to be nauseous now. Most girls get it at the end."

The nurse wheeled in a table with a machine on it and several other things, including two straps, or belts. The nurse wheeled the table to the side of the bed where Tim had been standing when he took her hand. "Here is your fetal monitor," said the nurse. "Now you'll have to lie down." Sheila lay back. The nurse pulled up her nightgown above her breasts and rubbed Sheila's body with something wet. She took each of the belts and placed them around Sheila's belly. While the nurse was placing the belts, Sheila had another contraction. The nurse was kind enough to stop her work until the contraction was over. Sheila panted and found the contraction felt different than the others and caused her to try and arch her lower back away from the bed to try and relieve the pressure there. When the contraction was over the nurse said, "Now I'm going to have to ask you to lie very still. Every movement you make shows up and it interferes with what we're looking for." She smiled and left. Ever so carefully, Sheila turned her head to see the lights and noise and the paper coming out of the machine. What she saw reminded her of a brain wave device she had seen once in a film in her high school health class. When Sheila had the next contraction she tried very hard not to arch her back away from the bed, but at the height of the contraction she grabbed the bars and had to lift off. After the contraction she thought to herself that it was all right to have done it because the patterns on the chart seemed the same even though she had moved.

Tim came back and told Sheila she looked different and he could see that a lot more progress had been made. He couldn't come close to her to hold her hand again because the table was in the way. Tim stayed behind it and timed her contractions.

The nurse came back wheeling a pole with a container hanging from the top of it. She maneuvered it up the side of the bed that was close to the wall and not only attached a needle to the vein on Sheila's hand but also taped and wrapped her entire hand to a wooden board. Sheila had two more contractions while the intravenous drip was being set up. "Now we should really get moving," the nurse told Tim with a wink when she left the room.

Sheila's next contraction came on quite suddenly and so strongly that Sheila was not able to keep control with her breathing. She yelled out a few times and clenched her teeth the rest of the time. When the contraction was over Sheila felt very frightened, and Tim looked frightened, too. He felt for Sheila's toes under the sheet and told her she was probably not very relaxed. He told her he would count out loud the seconds of the next contraction and that maybe this would help her. Sheila was very frightened of the next contraction starting and made a false start at the breathing, and Tim began counting in anticipation. Soon after they stopped, the real contraction came, and Sheila was able to breathe through most of it although at the end she had to clench her teeth and squeeze the bed bars again.

The nurse came back and checked the strip chart on the fetal monitor and made an adjustment to the intravenous drip. She asked Tim to try not to lean against the table where the monitor was. She left the room for a moment and came back with a chair for him to sit on, then left again.

Sheila had three more contractions and at the end of the third she began to cry. Tim rose to his feet and asked her what was the matter. "My back," sobbed Sheila. "I can't stand the pain. Get the nurse." Tim left to find the nurse. Sheila had another contraction and this time didn't bother to do a breathing exercise at all but just squirmed around the bed, squeezing the bars and keeping her mouth closed trying to keep from screaming. Her eyes were filled with tears, and she felt very ashamed.

The nurse and Tim came in, and Sheila began to explain how she felt. The nurse said understandingly, "We can do something for that. We'll give her something to take the edge off," she told Tim.

Sheila had another contraction during which she did a little breathing and a little yelling. The resident doctor she'd seen earlier came in and looked at her face. "Why so worried?" he said. Then he held out his hand onto which the nurse put a sterile glove. He examined Sheila and said, "Good." Then he gave the nurse some instructions. The nurse left, came back, and made an injection into the intravenous tubing. Sheila immediately had another contraction but was surprised to notice no difference in sensation so she squirmed around the bed a lot and gritted her teeth. "You can't be moving around so much," the nurse told Sheila while eyeing the fetal monitor printout. "Do your breathing."

Tim worked hard helping Sheila to keep up her breathing and she was able to complete most of her next four contractions without much squirming, gritting, or grabbing. She decided the medication must be working. She certainly felt more sleepy in between contractions. Tim also reported to her that her contractions were coming closer together and lasting longer. "No kidding," said Sheila.

When the nurse came in to check the monitor next time Sheila asked when her doctor would be coming. "You're not that far along yet," the nurse answered. "But he should be on his way."

When the nurse left, Sheila told Tim she was depressed that the nurse had said she was not very far along. The next half hour of contractions were very painful. After the last one she began to cry again. "I don't know how much more of this I can take," Sheila told Tim.

The nurse came in to check the monitor and Tim asked her if there wasn't anything more that could be done for Sheila's pain. "It's too early to give her anything stronger," the nurse told him. "You'll have to wait till her doctor comes." The nurse adjusted the intravenous drip again.

Sheila and Tim were quite unhappy during the next hour. It seemed harder and harder to keep on top of the contractions with the breathing. Sheila ached to turn over, but the belts seemed so heavy on her belly. She felt as if the feeling would last forever.

Sheila brightened when the doctor arrived. He came in quickly, and Sheila thought it was a good sign. "How are we?" he asked her.

"It's more painful than I thought," Sheila told him.

"It always is," he said. "I've decided on an epidural." Sheila knew that was a kind of local anesthetic and was happy she could still be awake for the birth. Her doctor held out his hand for a glove and examined Sheila.

"How far along am I?" asked Sheila.

"Oh, about six centimeters," said the doctor.

Sheila found it hard to believe she was only a little more than half dilated. "How much longer do you think it will be?" she asked him anxiously.

"There's no telling. I'd like to have you delivered soon, before infection sets in," he told her. "There's an increased chance of infection because her membranes ruptured so long ago," he told Tim. He gave the nurse some instructions, and they both left. The nurse came back and adjusted the intravenous drip, then inserted another injection.

"What are you doing?" Tim asked.

"Just my job," replied the nurse. "Remember yours is to time those contractions," she added with a smile.

The next hour seemed like forever to Sheila. It seemed as if everything was out of control; at the same time everything seemed slower. Tim left his chair and leaned near the table anyway and began to breathe along with Sheila and rub her feet. They got through two whole contractions with just breathing, but the rest were combinations of breathing and yelling.

Tim noticed the next time the nurse checked the monitor she looked concerned. She came back soon after with what looked like some plugs. The doctor came back this time, too. "We'll have to do some internal monitoring to check further," the doctor said. A plug or two was inserted up Sheila's vagina and something was taped to her leg.

Sheila kept screaming, "Ouch, ooh," while the doctor asked her to keep still. After about five minutes the nurse left, carrying something. Sheila became more frightened and yelled through her next contraction. "We'll take care of things soon," the doctor told her. He asked Tim if he could use his chair. "I'll be staying with your wife from here on in," he told Tim.

"Is there anything wrong?" Tim asked.

"No cause for alarm yet," the doctor said. "I'll tell you as soon as we know what's happening." He eyed the monitor from the chair and left it every few minutes to adjust something on the intravenous set-up. "We might be experiencing some fetal distress," he said at one point. "Let's try this." Suddenly he was lifting Sheila and turning her on her side.

Sheila couldn't believe she was being moved. *It's what I've been wanting all along,* she thought to herself. "Thank you, doctor,"

she told him several times. Sheila noticed that her back pain sub-
sided somewhat. The next contraction was still painful but instead
of yelling Sheila just sobbed into her pillow while biting it.

The nurse came back and said, "I have the lab report." The doctor
read it. He turned off the intravenous drip and stared at the fetal
monitor. It seemed to Sheila that everything was so quiet except
for the noise of the machine and except during her contractions,
after which she couldn't believe the sounds that had come out of
her. In between contractions she felt as if she had never been so
sad in her life. She no longer wanted to see Tim and was hoping
he couldn't see her.

The doctor cleared his throat. "We'll have to take steps now to
terminate the labor by operative intervention," he announced.

"Does that mean a cesarean?" Sheila heard Tim asking incredulously.

"I'm afraid so," answered the doctor. Sheila heard their voices,
but they seemed to come from a long distance. The doctor said Tim
would have to sign something.

"Will I get a shot to put me to sleep?" Sheila asked wearily.

"Of course," said the doctor. "I wouldn't want you to feel the
operation."

Sheila felt happy. During the next contraction she yelled a lot
and kept thinking. "This is the last one I'll feel." But she felt a
few more until people started moving her and giving her the injection. She remembered seeing Tim sheepishly wave to her and
leave the room looking very white, and she remembered feeling
nauseous again, and then a growing blackness.

Sheila thought she must be waking up in the operating room.
The doctor said something to her. She opened her mouth to reply,
but the sound from her body felt so painful that she went back to
sleep.

Sheila woke up again and there was Tim looking down at her.
"*So the operation must be over,*" she thought. She meant to ask
Tim if the baby was a boy or a girl but she dozed off.

When she woke up again, a nurse was saying, "Wake up, Mrs.
Willis. Can you use your bed pan?"

Sheila smiled. She tried to move her leg and felt excruciating
pain in her belly. She winced and fell back to sleep.

Sheila woke up in a room, and this time she was determined to
stay awake. She remembered someone telling her she'd had a son.
She remembered her labor and couldn't believe she could be lying

so still now. When she tried to move her hand she felt pain, so she didn't move again. She did move her eyes and saw an intravenous drip beside her.

She slept and woke up again, on and off. Sometimes a nurse would wake her to wash her or take her temperature. Her doctor came by and congratulated her. She smiled. He began talking about a "neat incision" and how she could "still wear a bikini." Sheila didn't tell him that she had never worn a bikini anyway.

The worst part about waking up was the pain. It felt as if she couldn't move anything without feeling pain. Once she tried to cough and her belly shook with such pain she spent a long time swallowing to prevent more coughs from coming up.

The best part about waking up was the time a nurse was standing over her holding a baby. Sheila realized it was hers. The nurse lay the baby next to Sheila and placed Sheila's arm around the tiny bundle. She felt her heart beating strongly. The baby was really moving his face. "Is it really a boy?" she asked the nurse. Sheila barely recognized the scratchy voice as her own.

"Of course," said the nurse. "But don't you go unwrapping him."

Sheila watched him beside her for many minutes. She realized the nurse was standing there to see that she didn't drop him. Then the nurse said her son had to go back to the nursery to be fed. Sheila felt jealous.

Another time when she was awake, a nurse told her she had to get up and walk to the bathroom. Sheila felt she must be dreaming. "You must be kidding," she said.

"All post-ops must be out of bed the day after surgery," the nurse told her. Then she added, "Don't worry, I'll help you." The nurse began moving Sheila to a sitting position at the edge of the bed. Sheila heard herself grunting with every move. The worst pain was near where her stitches must be. Sheila thought of the top edge of a bikini bottom cutting into her. When she was sitting at the edge of the bed the nurse put Sheila's slippers on her, placed her hands around the intravenous pole, and told her to stand up. Sheila's mind and body rebelled, and she made no effort to stand. Tears filled her eyes.

The nurse said, "Here, I'll help you." Slowly she lifted Sheila to standing. Suddenly she was really standing. It seemed as if the combined weight of her body and mind was on her incision. The pain burned her. She felt blood come out of her.

"I'm bleeding," Sheila told the nurse.

"Don't worry, your uterus is contracting. That's what this does," the nurse explained, pointing to the intravenous. "Now walk."

Sheila found she could move by sliding her feet slowly along the ground. She was hunched over, leaning against the pole on wheels, pushing it slowly ahead of her. "Very good," the nurse repeated in the high-pitched voice she had heard her sister-in-law use when her niece was learning to walk.

All Sheila could hear was the sound of her slippers sliding on the shiny floor. She became conscious for the first time that she had roommates. She knew they were all watching her. She estimated it took her about five to seven minutes to reach the bathroom, which was some thirty feet away.

The nurse pulled down Sheila's sanitary pad and helped her sit on the toilet. The pain shifted from her incision to her urethra. She tried to urinate but only a trickle came out. "I hope we don't have to put back the catheter," said the nurse. "You should be able to void yourself now." Sheila thought of the pain just to walk to the bathroom, the pain to urinate. The nurse seemed to sense her concern. "You can use the bedpan for the rest of today," she told Sheila. "Oh, thank you," Sheila said, trying to show her gratitude. The nurse helped Sheila stand up, and she felt that big weighty pain again. She moved back to her bed at what seemed an even slower pace because now she felt terribly weak. She grabbed the pole tightly. It was a long, painful process getting back to a reclining position. The nurse left. Sheila felt the nurse should have said something like, "I'm proud of you." She felt deeply humiliated and wished she had asked the nurse to pull the sheet up to her chin.

Later the nurse woke Sheila up and helped her comb her hair for visiting hours. Tim came. He kissed her and asked how she was feeling and how she liked the flowers. Sheila had to admit she hadn't noticed them. She told him how cute the baby was when they had brought him in. He said he knew because he had seen him through the nursery window. Sheila said she felt the most helpless she had ever been in her life. Tim said their family and friends had agreed she should just be happy to have a healthy baby. He said her mother was looking forward to visiting tomorrow. Sheila was glad he hadn't let her mother visit this time, because she looked and felt so terrible. She was sure tomorrow she'd feel much better.

And she was right. When the nurse woke her in the morning to take her temperature and told her she could start to eat some foods today, Sheila actually felt hungry. She tried to figure out how many days it had been since she had eaten food.

At ten o'clock they brought the baby to feed. They helped her to slowly sit up and she hardly felt the pain because she couldn't wait to hold the baby. They gave her a bottle. It was then she remembered that she had been thinking of breastfeeding. That seemed so long ago and, besides, she figured, her milk had probably dried up before it had even come in. The baby seemed eager to take the bottle. The nurse helped her burp the baby. Sheila vowed she would never prop the bottle and always hold her son close to her.

After they took the baby away, Sheila began to talk with the other women in the room. Of the four, three had had cesareans. The one who hadn't told them they should all be grateful for the fetal monitor. The woman moved around so easily. Then Sheila noticed that the two other women were moving around, too. She commented on it, and they assured her that soon she would be up and around.

One day Sheila realized how far she was progressing when one of her roommates left and another new mother was brought down to take her bed. The woman slept and moaned for about a day, and Sheila wondered if she had been like that, too. Sometimes Sheila looked down at her flattening belly to convince herself she was no longer pregnant. It seemed hard to make the transition in her mind, as if there were some missing pieces. Sheila also was disappointed that she hardly saw the baby during her hospital stay. On the third night she had developed a low-grade fever which recurred the next evening, and hospital rules stated that a mother couldn't have her baby to feed unless her temperature was normal for twenty-four hours. Sheila had laughed an embarrassed laugh when she had pointed out the wrong baby in the nursery to a visitor.

When the fever disappeared, Sheila's doctor told her she was making such a speedy recovery that she could leave on the sixth day even though he preferred to keep patients hospitalized a week. This lifted Sheila's spirits because she had always thought of herself as a strong person. On the sixth day Sheila gave the nurse some new baby clothes to dress her son. Tim came up to the room to get her. She began to walk to the nursery to get the baby, but a hospital volunteer brought a wheelchair and told her she must sit in it until they reached the exit. This reminded Sheila of the night she had entered the hospital. She seemed a whole different person then. "Now I'm a mother," Sheila told herself proudly. Another volunteer carried the baby in the elevator and told Sheila she could have him when she left the building. Sheila wondered if Tim was anxious to get his hands on the baby for the first time.

At the door Sheila stood up and the volunteer handed her the baby. Suddenly she felt afraid. But Tim held her arm and steered her to the waiting car. As he opened the door in a grand gesture to allow her to take her seat, Sheila saw a flash from a movie or a magazine picture advertisement. She couldn't remember where she had seen it. "*The happy American family,*" Sheila thought. She smiled. She felt strangely confused.

HOSPITAL PROCEDURES

What happened to Sheila happens to hundreds of birthing women each day in this country's hospitals. At their most life-giving moments women are subject to a barrage of mistreatment that may cause emotional degradation and present serious hazards to the well-being of both mother and baby. Many procedures which were originally developed to deal with isolated cases of pathology have become the rule for all normal women and babies. As couples become increasingly aware of these procedures and the research on their possible side effects, it is no wonder that more women are staying home to have their babies.

These are just some of the routine hospital procedures surrounding birth that may be at best unnecessary and at worst harmful. First, some specific interventions will be discussed, and then larger issues like electronic fetal monitoring and cesareans will be discussed.

The Prep

When a woman is admitted to the hospital her pubic hair may be shaved, an enema may be administered, and an intravenous (IV) needle will be inserted into her vein. What are the pros and cons of these procedures?

Some doctors say they no longer shave all the pubic hair, they just do a "mini-prep," which means some of the pubic hair is shaved. They say this practice helps them to see better. But even the thickest hair is separated as the baby's head pushes through the vagina. Doctors also say that the baby can pick up an infection when it passes by the pubic hair. But in the hospital a woman's perineum may be bathed in antiseptic solution anyway. Studies published in *Obstetrics and Gynecology* as early as 1964 and 1965 showed that, if anything, infection was slightly higher among shaved women due to razor cuts and abrasions. Many women fear receiving such cuts, and the hair growing back is uncomfortable and itchy. Shaving may also rob the mother of protection for her genitals that the hair was originally intended to provide.

The medical reason for the enema is that impacted feces can impede the passage of the baby's head down and out of the mother's body. A woman who has not moved her bowels for several days would probably be wise to accept an enema, but if she will be uncomfortable feeling its effect during the throes of powerful contractions she can purchase an enema at a drug store and administer it to herself in early labor in the comfort of her own bathroom. Sometimes an enema has a therapeutic effect, shaking up a dormant labor, and it is certainly safer than going right away for a strong drug to augment labor. Any mother who doesn't have an enema should be aware of the possibility of expelling fecal matter while pushing out the baby, but nurses are prepared for this possibility and simply wipe it away.

The IV

As for the IV, doctors usually offer two main reasons why it is given. The first is that the mother needs fluid and energy for labor. This is true, but wouldn't, for example, a half gallon of apple juice sipped through labor accomplish the same purpose? Doctors usually respond at this point that mothers in labor should not eat and drink in case they need a general anesthetic for an emergency cesarean, and there is a danger of vomiting after general anesthesia and aspirating the vomitus. In spite of the fact that surgeons use a nasogastric tube to administer the anesthetic, which separates the trachea from the esophagus, and in spite of speculation on what deprivation of real food for up to twenty-four hours might do to uterine function (athletes know that if they don't eat energy foods their body parts don't come through for them), doctors still stress the danger of this potential occurrence.

The second reason for the IV that is given is that if the mother needs a blood transfusion, there already is an open vein, so this saves times in attaching a needle for the transfusion. This, in spite of the fact that alternatives for transfusion are tried with increasing frequency because of the risk of contracting Acquired Immune Deficiency Syndrome virus from blood transfusion. The reasons given for the IV are good examples of what Suzanne Arms has termed the practice of "just-in-case obstetrics."

Confinement to Bed

This is an example of a procedure which was originally introduced for a specific medical reason and now may be required routinely. Earlier in the century, when most women who had hospital births were heavily medicated during labor, it would have been dangerous for them to move about. In fact sometimes a tent was placed over the hospital bed to prevent the woman from leaving. If these women had gotten out of bed there was a good chance they would have fallen and seriously injured themselves or their babies. But if a woman is not medicated, why confine her to bed?

The upright posture actually speeds up her labor by allowing gravity to help the baby's head move further down in the pelvis. Also, if the mother is upright and engaged in activity she is not concentrating on the discomfort of her labor, so she has less pain. The position also decreases maternal effort. Research has shown that contractions are more intense and efficient (they dilate the cervix more) when a woman is standing. A study published in 1984 in the *British Journal of Obstetrics & Gynecology* found that women who walked more than 60 percent of the time during their labor had shorter first and second (pushing) stages of labor than women who stayed in bed. Lying down not only slows down body processes, but the weight of the baby and the uterus on the main blood vessels that run down the back can actually compromise the oxygen supply to the baby. Dr. Roberto Caldeyro-Barcia, a past president of the International Confederation of Obstetricians and Gynecologists who studies the effects of obstetric interferences, has found that lying down causes the mother's blood pressure to drop, which can lead to fetal asphyxia, because the uterus is compressing the aorta and the inferior vena cava. Another side effect is muscle weakness.

Artificial Rupture of the Bag of Waters

If the bag of amniotic fluid has not broken naturally by the time the woman comes to the hospital (the normal time for the bag to break is during transition, at the end of labor), many doctors will prick the bag with a knitting needle-like prong to cause the flow. This procedure, they tell the woman, will speed up her labor. Contractions usually do come at a faster and stronger pace after rupture. But artificial rupture does not come without its hazards.

Besides making the contractions more difficult for some women to control when they suddenly increase in strength, the absence of the bag of waters can have life-threatening effects on the baby. Dr. Caldeyro-Barcia has found that the amniotic fluid is important as a cushion for the baby during labor contractions and that the absence of the fluid can cause brain deformation, with possible hemorrhage and even death, as the baby's now unprotected head continually pounds on the cervix. Dr. Caldeyro-Barcia states, "The question is whether it is worthwhile to reduce labor by thirty to forty minutes at the expense of all the deformation and possible damage to the head of the fetus." If the bag of waters is left to rupture naturally, closer to the time of birth, the fetus appears better able to tolerate the pressure.

Moving From Labor Bed To Delivery Table

Even those of us who grew up away from the farm know that if a cat is in labor you don't move her. If she's found her nice, quiet, dark, warm, safe place in the corner of your clothes closet, you don't move her out under the fluorescent lights so you can view the birth better. Yet we don't usually show a human mother the same respect by allowing her to give birth in the same bed she labored in. Jostling a mother about at a time when she is in hardest labor, speeding her down a hallway and shaking her up some more to put her on a narrow high table as her baby's head is about to emerge are most inconsiderate actions. The fast ride in the hallway and the high position of the narrow table cause some mothers to fear the baby will fall out onto the floor. Also, the sight of an equipped hospital delivery room is not conducive to a relaxed, enjoyable childbirth. Niles Newton, Ph.D., of Northwestern University Medical School's Psychiatry Department, found that more rat pups died when their mothers were moved at the time of birth.

Lithotomy Position

The lithotomy position means the woman is flat on her back, with her legs raised, separated, and strapped into metal stirrups. Sometimes her hands are tied down as well. For an awake mother, intent on actively participating in her child's birth, the position is a degradation.

The lithotomy position is clearly for the convenience of the person viewing the birth and has nothing whatsoever to do with comfort, safety, or health of the mother or baby. It is, in fact, the worst possible birth position for mother and baby. It adversely affects the mother's blood pressure, comfort, and intensity of contractions. It works against gravity in pushing out the baby. Thus other obstetrical interference, such as drugs, forceps, and episiotomy, to name a few, must be employed to extract the baby. These in turn carry with them their own side effects. The lithotomy position may be seen as the original causative factor for most of the damage caused by birth injuries.

Delaying Birth

Birth can be delayed by medication or by forcing the mother to cross her legs or by having a nurse actually hold the head in. It is widely known that there is a good chance that delaying birth in these ways may result in a brain-damaged baby. Yet occasionally these procedures are still employed if the doctor is on his way to the delivery but has not yet arrived. Or, the procedure may be used for clearly nonmedical reasons. The decade was ushered in, according to newspaper reports, with a three-city race for first baby of the '80s. Speaking of a birth about to occur in the last minutes before midnight Dec. 31, 1979, a Chicago hospital's administrative supervisor was quoted as saying, "We were holding her head back, trying to get the title!"

Episiotomy

An episiotomy is a cut that most doctors make at the base of the woman's vagina. They say they make it to widen the opening so the baby's head can fit through and so the head doesn't tear the woman in an uncontrolled direction. Episiotomy is so routine in this country that its occurrence is discussed with the same acceptance as the appearance of the baby's head. Concerned childbirth educators debate whether the baby's head presses the mother's nerve endings sufficiently to squeeze out sensation so that an injection of a painkiller before an episiotomy is not necessary. Concerned doctors discuss the merits of the different directions of making the cut. Weeks after delivery, women complain about their stitches more vociferously than about their whole labors. The endearing term "husband's knot" has been coined by winking obstetricians to describe that extra stitch given to unsuspecting mothers when sewing up the episiotomy. The "husband's knot" makes her "like a virgin again" so her husband will have "more fun," though she'll be in considerable pain.

Actually, an episiotomy causes bleeding which, when added to the normal blood loss after the birth of a baby, may amount to enough to put the woman into shock. An episiotomy also increases the chance of infection and other obstetrical interference such as drugs. Cutting violates a woman's body. No one likes to have surgery performed, however minor, unless it is necessary. Yet episiotomy is performed routinely in this country while the episiotomy rate in almost every other country of the world is considerably lower. Comparing episiotomy rates for doctors and for midwives, one finds the midwife rate much lower than the doctor rate, because slower delivery of the baby's head, nonlithotomy position, and use of warm compresses and perineal massage—all of which are more common with midwives—help prevent the need for episiotomy and help prevent tearing. A study on the first 4,000 births of the Frontier Nursing Service in Kentucky, where nurse-midwives attended women at home, reported the episiotomy rate at 0.4 percent.

Some doctors tell women their insides will fall through later in life if they don't have episiotomies now. Women truly concerned with this fallacy can tell their doctors they intend to do Kegel exercises (contracting and releasing the muscles of the pelvic floor) which help improve muscle tone at any time. British anthropologist and childbirth educator Sheila Kitzinger completed a research study for the National Childbirth Trust in 1981 in which she compared women who had had episiotomy with women who had torn. She found that "women who have had episiotomies with spontaneous vaginal deliveries experience more pain at the end of the first week after delivery than those who have had lacerations and are more likely to find it difficult to get into or maintain a position in which they can comfortably breastfeed. They are more likely to experience dyspareunia [pain on intercourse] and to have it longer than those who have had lacerations."

Two more recent studies have suggested that episiotomy actually causes tears. In a Belgian study, third-degree tears occurred in more women who had just had an episiotomy than women without one. In a study reported in 1986 from the University of Cincinnati Medical Center, third and fourth degree tears were found only in women who underwent episiotomy. And if the episiotomy was considered equal to a second degree laceration, women without episiotomy experienced fewer lacerations 78 percent of the time.

It is important to remember that the choice is not whether to tear or be cut. Without an episiotomy, in a low-stress physiological birth position, your perineum is likely to remain intact.

Forceps

It is easier for forceps to go in when an episiotomy is performed. Obstetrical textbooks discuss the evolution of these spoon-shaped pliers (their development and use were confined as a secret within one family of doctors for more than a hundred years), and they have saved countless babies' lives when immediate extraction was needed to rescue a troubled fetus who had to be born more quickly.

But today they are used up to 65 percent of the time in some American hospitals, although some have replaced their use with suction aspiration to extract the baby quickly. The increase in epidural anesthesia is another factor because being numb from the waist down gives a woman little control over the expulsive effort. Drugs is another factor which gives the woman little control over the expulsive effort. But most mothers are not made aware that forceps are responsible not only for distorted-looking faces and heads of newborns, but also hemorrhages and nerve damage of the brain which can cause other neurological impairment. It is also possible that forceps can cause internal damage to the mother.

Early clamping of the umbilical cord

This denies the infant not only up to 25 percent of the blood supply she or he is entitled to, but also a smooth transition from cord support to external support. Early clamping has also been linked with delayed placenta expulsion and retained placenta.

Speeding up the removal of the placenta

In the interest of clearing out the delivery room speedily to clean up for the lady waiting in the wings, different methods of hastily removing the placenta are employed, from pressing on the woman's belly to giving her *Pitocin* to actually tugging on the umbilical cord. Some women are told that if the placenta doesn't come out with the next scheduled contraction within about two to five minutes there is a problem. While it is true that a retained placenta or pieces of placenta can cause infection or hemorrhage, procedures like pulling on the umbilical cord can actually cause the retained pieces and subsequent infection and hemorrhage. It is probably normal in most cases, provided there is no hemorrhage or other sign of problem with the mother, for the placenta to take a while to come out, up to an hour or more. But what doctor in a hospital will wait around that long? Sometimes a so-called retained placenta has already been separated from the wall of the uterus and the woman must simply be helped to squat to push it out.

Separating the mother from her newborn

At most hospitals an awake mother is shown her newborn or permitted to hold her a little while, but the baby is eventually taken away to a baby warmer for a newborn exam or a stay in the nursery. A federal government panel has cautioned that radiant warmers expose newborns to the risk of hyperthermia, which may result in death or permanent neurological damage. Also, water loss increases when infants are placed under radiant warmers, and first-degree burns have been attributed to the warmers heating plastic-lined disposable diapers. Questions on delayed effects of exposure to infared radiation on newborns' eyes have been raised. Most mothers would rather warm their newborn on their own bodies (98.6°), with a blanket being placed over them both, if necessary, and the newborn exam occurring between her legs. This may necessitate raising the delivery room thermostat, which is usually kept lower for the comfort of the staff, not keeping the needs of a newborn in mind.

Separating a baby from its mother at any time after birth not only may interfere with a good start in breastfeeding but also interrupts with the bonding that is the start of a good mother-child relationship. Bonding is not something that can be scheduled in a one-hour period, as some hospitals have done, but is an on-going process of people getting to know and be responsive to each other. Certainly the administration of eye drops to all newborns immediately after birth, because an occasional mother could have gonorrhea, interferes with the ability of newborns to see their parents. As for the rest of family bonding, it is an improvement at some hospitals to have sibling visitation, but the natural, gradual acceptance of the newborn that occurs in a home birth cannot be duplicated in a hospital.

Although more hospitals offer rooming-in of the baby, now that more women are breastfeeding, very few offer it for twenty-four hours. Or it may be limited to availability of certain rooms or situations, so not all mothers who want it can have it. Bringing the baby on a four-hour schedule is not conducive to successful breastfeeding, since most newborns want to nurse approximately every two hours. Delays and scheduling can prevent the onset of an adequate milk supply, since there is not adequate stimulation, and can cause painful engorgement once the milk does come in. Additionally, uncooperative nurses with misinformation may feed the baby formula without checking first on family allergies, or they may insist that the mother bottlefeed the baby sugar water at each feeding time.

Drugs

There are other types of interventions that could be debated, such as whether or not to suction mucus from the baby's respiratory tract or let the newborn negotiate his or her own mucus. But these issues are relatively mild compared to major issues of concern that have of late defined hospitalized birth in the United States. Issues like drugs, malpractice, electronic fetal monitoring, and the rise in cesareans are interconnected and have far-reaching implications.

It is a myth that fewer drugs are being given now that more women take natural childbirth classes. Maybe more women are learning about a drug-free birth in their childbirth classes, but since the cesarean rate has increased at least 500 percent in twenty years, even if more women have a local anesthetic so they can remain awake for their operation, still more drugs are being given. The amount of labor augmentation has also increased; in one unpublished survey, at least three-fourths of all women at some city hospitals were being given *Pitocin* during labor. And at least one old drug is making a comeback: scopolamine, whose use in labor had been on the downswing, is becoming more popular again.

It is not necessary to review here all the drugs that may be given in labor and their potential side-effects to the mother and baby. This information should be forthcoming to the mother. She may look it up in the library in the *Physicians Desk Reference,* a book published for physicians with prescribing information from the drug companies including potential side-effects. This information is also included in the "package insert" of drugs. So, if a mother has trouble finding this book, she can read the physician's or the pharmacist's copy. Some drugs you may want to look up are *Demerol* and *Pitocin,* which are used during labor, and "caine" drugs like *Lidocaine* and *Marcaine* that are used in epidural anesthesia at the end of labor. *Pitocin,* for example, may be given at such a pace that the artificially induced contractions come crashingly fast, leaving little "breather space" in between for the baby's heart rate to return to normal. Or the tumultuous contractions may cause uterine rupture or premature separation of the placenta. These possibilities should be discussed with the mother before the drug is given to comply with the doctrine of informed consent. In New York State a doctor or midwife must inform the mother of any potential side-effects to herself or her baby of any drug that is prescribed for her during pregnancy, labor, or birth. This law was introduced due to the persistence of a New York mother whose son was brain-damaged by *Pitocin.* Of course, there is a high rate of noncompliance with this law, but mothers must be vigilant.

Mothers should also ask what alternatives are available. A 1985 study at an Army Medical Center in California reported that nipple stimulation is a nondrug way to initiate labor contractions, because it causes the release of oxytocin from the pituitary gland. (*Pitocin,* a synthetic hormone, was developed to simulate oxytocin.)

The American Academy of Pediatrics' Committee on Drugs has stated that there is no drug that has been proven safe for the unborn. The Food and Drug Administration has not tested most drugs on the market for pregnancy safety (partly because it is not ethical to give drugs to an experimental group of pregnant women to see what, if anything, happens to their fetuses). Most drugs a mother ingests do pass through the umbilical cord and the placenta to the fetus. It is not unusual for a drugged baby to be born sluggish and to be slow in taking its first breath. Very long delays in initiating respiration usually result in brain damage. A mother doesn't always realize that, although the effect the drug has on her is often gone in a matter of hours, since the liver and kidneys detoxify her system, the newborn's system doesn't operate so efficiently. And the immature brain stores the drugs for a week or longer, affecting the baby's behavior. How many mothers would be willing to withstand temporary pain if they had the full information? A drugged baby and mother also have their bonding impulses suppressed.

Mothers should also consider side-effects that may not be reported because they are not a direct effect of the drug being administered. Consider, for example, that if *Pitocin* makes contractions unnaturally strong, the mother is more likely to ask for and receive a pain-killing drug. In some hospitals, a *Pitocin-Demerol-Pitocin* cycle is observed. Since the *Demerol* may have a slowing effect on uterine contractions, the mother may need more *Pitocin* to speed up labor again. But after more *Pitocin* is given, she will need more *Demerol,* and on and on.

In other countries, drugs for birthing women are kept to a minimum or not given at all. The support a woman receives from her midwife and husband is usually enough to prevent her from perceiving her discomfort as unbearable. But in this country, doctors don't discourage or they actually encourage the use of drugs, since they themselves offer little or no emotional support as an alternative. Drugs are so widespread among women in labor that blue extremities on newborns, usually indicating oxygen deprivation, is thought normal by medical students. Gail Grogan, writing for her master's thesis at New York University, concluded that educating parents about the risks of drugs and unnecessary interventions not only results in healthier infants but also a more satisfying birth experience. The key, she says, is giving parents a choice in the matter.

Fetal Monitors

One area where there is less and less choice concerns electronic fetal monitoring. At most hospitals in the country, it is now routine for all laboring women, whether they have been labelled high risk or low risk. And there are no studies to point to when questioning the long-term effects of electronic monitoring. Women having babies in the hospital today *are* the experimental group! A routine procedure has been introduced on a national basis for all laboring women without demonstrated benefit first. This, in a medical culture where five Cleveland doctors had to travel to Guatemala, on grants from the Public Health Service plus two foundations, to publish a study in the *New England Journal of Medicine* in 1980 "suggesting" that women with a constant companion during labor got through it more easily![1] Where are the studies showing the safety and benefit of routine electronic fetal monitoring before it was instituted on such a widespread basis?

There are two types of electronic fetal monitoring. With external monitoring, two belts encircle the mother's abdomen. One picks up the intensity of the mother's contractions, the other the baby's heart rate. This information is transferred to a screen on a small box placed on a table next to the mother's labor bed. Or the information may be transferred to a central screening area near the nurses' station so many women in labor can be monitored at once. The information is also recorded on a printout, or strip chart, which, as one advertisement for an electronic monitor company tellingly announced, fits conveniently in the mother's chart in case it is needed in the future. With internal monitoring, an electrode which looks like a small corkscrew is inserted into the baby's scalp or other presenting part (necessitating the breaking of the bag of waters), and a wire lead is taped to the mother's thigh. The information from internal monitoring is also transferred to the TV screen-like recorder. The internal monitor is generally considered more accurate than the external.

Reported side-effects of electronic monitoring include the unseating of the husband from the machine's presence in the labor room, lack of uniformity in reading the results, a high rate of innaccuracy due, among other reasons, to malfunction (before a decision to do a cesarean based on an electronic monitor reading is reached, a fetal blood sample should have been taken, where a low pH would be a more accurate indicator of oxygen deprivation to the baby), and the medical attendants read the machine instead of talking to the laboring mother. Perhaps the most serious consequence of monitoring is that the woman is asked to lie down for an accurate reading. Thus its use may cause its justification. In other words, the prolonged supine position may effect the circulation of blood and oxygen to the baby, because the compression of the vena cava and aorta may effect circulation to the mother. Then, fetal distress may be reported, with the ironic question, "Aren't you glad you were on the fetal monitor?" Complications of internal monitoring include scalp abscesses, infections, hemorrhage, and even death to the fetus.

One of the more serious considerations in assessing the effect of routine electronic fetal monitoring is the use of ultrasound. Ultrasound as a diagnostic tool for pregnant women on a large-scale basis is also relatively recent. There are three main ways that pregnant women may be routinely exposed to ultrasound. One is by sonograms, ultrasonic "pictures" of the fetus which may be ordered throughout the pregnancy as a way to view the size or development of the fetus. Sonograms are also required in connection with amniocentesis, so the baby isn't stuck by the needle when amniotic fluid is withdrawn. Another is by the doppler, the device used routinely during prenatal care to scan the mother's belly and amplify the baby's heart beat. The third is through electronic monitoring during labor, which has already been described. These last two types of heart-rate monitoring have replaced the fetoscope, a specially shaped stethoscope that was previously used to auscultate the baby's heart rate without ultrasound.

Additionally, some women are exposed to ultrasound before they actually go into labor, by stress tests or nonstress tests that some doctors order if the mother goes past her estimated due date. In these tests, the mothers are sent to the hospital and placed on the electronic monitor (lying down, of course, which induces stress), and the baby's heart rate is recorded, with or without the addition of *Pitocin* to cause contractions.

The problem is that we don't yet know if ultrasound used diagnostically during pregnancy has long-term effects. Still, some doctors are quick to state, "Don't worry about it; it's only sound waves." This same casual attitude was also expressed when X-radiation was introduced as a diagnostic tool and used for many purposes, from X-raying children's feet in a shoe store to treating swollen glands and acne. Animal studies have revealed delayed neuromuscular development, altered emotional behavior, EEG changes, anomalies, and decreased survival with ultrasound. Dr. D. Liebeskind at Albert Einstein Medical College in New York has demonstrated DNA changes in cells exposed to ultrasound in a laboratory setting.[2] Some Canadian studies on human babies exposed to ultrasound in utero suggest slight hearing loss or slightly lower birth weight. This may not seem like much, but the point is that ultrasound does cause changes. Women's health advocate Doris Haire questions the effect of ultrasound on the ova of female fetuses.[3] Since girls are born with all their eggs, we may not know until the next generation, when our daughters have babies, whether a higher percentage of offspring born to women who were exposed to ultrasound when they were in utero have a particular abnormality. We just don't know. If it is the age of the baby that is ever shown to be critical, then early sonograms may be implicated. If it is the strength of frequency that is critical, the doppler may be implicated, since it uses high frequency. And if it is the length of exposure, electronic monitoring during labor may be implicated, since the belt may be on the mother for ten or more hours during labor.

Jay Hathaway, a director of the American Academy of Husband-Coached Childbirth, has even questioned the use of the word "ultrasound." He asks, "Would anyone call nuclear radiation ultralight? Ultrasound is not sound, *i.e.,* vibration in the audible range. It is so far above the audible range. . . . [T]his new radiation is even higher in frequency than the AM radio band, a long way above sound."[4] Maybe that is why some mothers report their babies "jump" during a sonogram.

The small amount of research which has appeared in the United States has been concerned mostly with the benefits of electronic fetal monitoring during labor. Early research was conducted by Dr. Albert Haverkamp at Denver General Hospital.[5] In his study, hundreds of high-risk women were attached to the internal electronic monitor. In half the women, the machine was turned off, and a nurse auscultated the baby's heart rate with a fetoscope. In the machine-monitored group, there were two and a half times more cesareans, a 13.2 percent infection rate compared to only 3.4 percent of the nurse-monitored women, and five machine-monitored babies were in need of resuscitation two minutes after birth, while none of the nurse-monitored babies needed help to breathe.

Soon after, Drs. David Banta and Stephen Thacker were commissioned by the federal government to research the benefits, particularly cost benefits, of electronic fetal monitoring. In a report with nearly 300 references, they concluded that for most childbearing women, the risks of electronic monitoring exceed the benefits and that those risks were costing Americans hundreds of millions of dollars a year.[6] Several months later a government-appointed task force suggested that electronic fetal monitoring should not be used on a routine basis and that it should be "strongly considered" only in high-risk pregnancies.

More recently, a 1986 study reported in the *New England Journal of Medicine* reviewed nearly 35,000 births in Dallas and found no improvement in fetal outcome from monitoring, even though twice as many cesareans were performed in the universally monitored group. The authors concluded that not all pregnancies, particularly not low-risk ones, need continuous electronic monitoring. Even if irregular heart rates were shown, the babies were actually fine.[7]

In spite of this research, routine electronic monitoring of all pregnant women persists. Why this is so appears to be tied up in broader issues like the increase in malpractice suits of obstetricians. The strip chart is written, permanent proof that the woman was monitored during labor. If the physician is sued, he can produce evidence that the woman was monitored, even if he didn't show up until the delivery. Without the strip chart, he would have to rely on nurses' notes from fetoscope auscultation, which is not considered state-of-the-art.

Surgery

And research for the federal government by Helen Marieskind has shown that fear of malpractice suits is the number one reason doctors perform cesareans as frequently as they do. If something is wrong with the baby and a cesarean has been performed, a jury may feel that the doctor did all he could. But if something is wrong with the baby and a cesarean hasn't been performed, the first question a jury may ask is "Why didn't he do a cesarean?"

Other reasons Marieskind found for the rise in cesareans include repeat cesareans, although recent research has shown the risk of rupture to the previous cesarean's uterine scar to be less than the risk of repeat major surgery, and reliance on the electronic fetal monitor as the tool by which doctors make decisions. In addition to the appearance of so-called fetal distress, she also found an increase in diagnosis of dystocia ("failure to progress," a subjective concept) and "CPD" (cephalopelvic disproportion) as reasons for cesarean. If a woman is flat on her back, with no upright posture to allow spreading of the pelvic outlet and molding of the baby's head, how can we ever know if she had CPD?

Indeed, recent statistics show that, nationally, 22.7 percent of all babies are born by cesarean.[8] At some major teaching hospitals, the rate passes 30 percent. In comparison with other developed countries, the United States is a leader in cesareans, with Canada a close second; in many other countries the rate is still under 10 percent. Does this mean that one in three or four of us is incapable of delivering vaginally?

The risks to the mother and baby from cesarean are well documented, yet most mothers are not informed that a cesarean section is major surgery. With major surgery, there is always the possibility that the anesthetic will be improperly administered, and there is an increased likelihood of hemorrhage and infection. In one Rhode Island study two doctors compared maternal death rates and found a risk factor twenty-six times greater for cesareans than for vaginal deliveries.[9] Almost all women have severe pain and gas problems. For the baby, serious problems center around respiratory distress and lung problems and jaundice and drug effects.

Still, most doctors justify the high cesarean rate, saying the surgery is "safe." A few influential obstetricians have even suggested universal cesareans! Most point to the reduction in neonatal mortality as a result of increased cesareans.

However, Drs. Kieran O'Driscoll and Michael Foley questioned this common assumption in a study published in 1983. Citing nearly 109,000 births at the National Maternity Hospital in Dublin from 1965 to 1980, they noted that in their country the mortality rate improved 60 percent while the cesarean rate remained virtually constant at around 4 percent.[10] Although perinatal mortality improved 50 percent in the United States at a time when the cesarean rate increased 300 percent, the authors concluded, "These results do not support the contention that the expansion in cesarean birth rates has contributed significantly to reduced perinatal mortality in recent years."[10]

In spite of this, doctors show no sign of holding back on the decision to order surgery. Many doctors routinely do cesareans for all breech presentations, although a 1981 study from Canada showed breech babies born vaginally scored the same or better on standard neonatal tests than breech babies delivered by cesarean.[11] The infants were followed up to eight years after birth, and no difference in subsequent development was found.

Other reasons given for necessary cesareans are also being questioned. In 1982 a pregnant woman in Jackson, Michigan was ordered by the local court to enter the hospital and undergo a cesarean. Instead she went into hiding and gave birth to a healthy 9 lb. 3 oz. boy without surgery. Doctors had testified that the cesarean was required because the mother had placenta previa, a low-lying placenta which partially or totally covers the cervix.

The old maxim, "Once a cesarean, always a cesarean," has also been questioned. Vaginal birth after cesarean (VBAC) has now

been endorsed by the American College of Obstetricians and Gynecologists. But although the percentage of VBAC has more than
doubled since 1970, over 90 percent of previously sectioned mothers
have a repeat cesarean. There is still a great fear that the uterine
scar from the previous cesarean will tear, although this rarely
happens. Some observers think that early cesarean support groups
had focused too much on making the cesarean a pleasant experience rather than aggressively attacking the reasons for their frequency.[12]

And Susan Doering of Johns Hopkins University conducted a
study in which she found that although births are spread randomly
around the clock, 80 percent of so-called emergency cesareans occurred during daylight hours, usually between one and five P.M.
Her finding suggests that obstetricians may choose to do a cesarean
when they simply don't want to wait into the night for the labor
to progress to its natural conclusion.[13]

Yet, home birth proponents are not against cesareans, or any
other intervention, when used for a good medical reason. They
object to the *routine* use, many times for teaching purposes, of
procedures that have been introduced for a specific medical condition of a specific mother or baby. An added problem is the snow-
ball effect, illustrated in the 1981 study published in *The Journal
of Family Practice* by Drs. Brody and Thompson. They point out
that each obstetrical intervention can't be considered in isolation
but must be seen as part of an interconnected system, where often
the side-effects of one procedure necessitate the introduction of
another procedure, and on and on.

Always, the risks and benefits of accepting a particular procedure
must be weighed against the risks and benefits of rejecting it. And
hospitalization itself, as a treatment for birth, is no exception.

CHAPTER 5

Doctor, Midwife, or Do-It-Yourself?

As the story goes, a man once said to Ina May, head midwife at the Farm, a spiritual community in Summertown, Tennessee, "Well, I don't know what we need midwives for. Childbirth is as natural as taking a shit. All you have to do is squat down and do it." To which Ina May is said to have replied, "Yes, but we are not called upon to make a turd breathe."

Every laboring mother and newborn baby are entitled to the care of a qualified birth attendant. Rejection of the hospital setting for normal birth should not be construed as rejection of sensible assistance in the person of a trained and experienced birth attendant. The presence of the baby's mother and father alone is not enough to make home birth safe and attractive in all cases.

Today some couples, forced to choose between an unattended home birth or an American-style hospital birth, opt to stay at home anyway. The woman is usually seeing an obstetrician for prenatal care and he becomes the hospital backup. Some obstetricians do not learn of the couple's plans until after the fact, especially if the doctor seems the type who would then refuse prenatal care, as many do. Usually the couple reads a lot and gains a relatively good textbook knowledge of normal labor and birth and the signs of abnormality. The father catches the baby and eventually clamps the umbilical cord with boiled shoelaces.

In other cases the woman chooses to remain totally alone. Pat Carter of Florida delivered nine of her own babies herself, refusing to let her husband be present, and wrote about her experiences in the underground classic, *Come Gently, Sweet Lucina*.[1] Her League of Liberated Women counted as its members only those women who "have borne at least one child on purpose without professional attendance." Some women give birth at home by mistake, usually because they are so relaxed that they don't recognize advanced labor for what it is.

And a new national organization devoted to do-it-yourself home birth parents has gained popularity. Formerly known as the Birth at Home League, the title of the group was changed to The New Nativity, more accurately reflecting its Christian outlook. Members of The New Nativity quote from biblical scripture to support their philosophy, stating that a man, as head of his home, should deliver his wife's baby, aided by strong religious conviction. The head of the group, Marilyn Moran, has written a delightful book, *Birth and the Dialogue of Love*, stressing the sensuality and sexuality of birth.

As a group, all these kinds of births are known as medically unattended home births. There is no known study on unattended home births *vs*. hospital deliveries, but it is not likely that the unattended home births would fare poorly. Birth is one area where things usually come out normally, even—or especially—when there is no outside interference.

With the exception of committed New Nativity parents, however, many couples who elect to do it themselves say that they would prefer to have a qualified attendant at the birth—it's just that they are unable to find one willing to come to the home. If the couple looked to a doctor or nurse-midwife for help, this refusal represents an abdication of professional responsibility on the part of organized medicine—those doctors who refuse to come to the home, knowing that the baby will be born there anyway, and those who refuse to give prenatal care. Doctors who refuse to give prenatal care are acting even more deplorably, since office checkups do not inconvenience them, as attending a birth at home might. Some say that if they gave prenatal care, the patient might think the doctors condone her plans and that by refusing it they hope to leave her no choice but to have her baby in the hospital.

Dr. John S. Miller, author of *Childbirth: A Manual for Expectant Parents,* thoughtfully admits, "I have reminded myself not to be shocked by the thought of a young mother and father willing to run a risk with their baby's life. Because, in a sense, I was willing to run the same risk in my refusal to go to their homes to deliver them. We all say we are interested in perinatal mortality, but only on our conditions—only when the patient is willing to submit to what we find convenient. If she is willing to come to us and be delivered by our method, then we are interested. . . . Solutions are so far in the future that we can only contemplate some halfway measure—changes which fill only partly those needs that the patients express to us by staying away."[2]

WHY HAVE A BIRTH ATTENDANT?

There are several reasons why it is better to have a birth attendant besides the parents present. The most important is that the birth attendant will be in a position to more readily recognize signs of complications, albeit rare, that may require emergency intervention or hospitalization. Anyone acting as a birth attendant should be familiar with the signs of premature separation of the placenta, placenta previa, fetal distress, a malpresentation such as hand first, a depressed newborn, and hemorrhage and be able to evaluate those signs in terms of emergency measures and possible hospitalization.

Even if the baby's father is as well read as a novice birth attendant or has been to a few births of friends, he cannot function well in a dual role if he must also be the emotional support of the baby's mother. Literally and figuratively, he cannot be at both ends of the woman at once, and both ends are equally important. Also, the father is emotionally involved in the birth of his child. A birth attendant who is not the father is capable of making an independent evaluation if there is anything that seems amiss. A third person can step back, be objective and detached, and come to a rational decision more easily.

A birth attendant is also someone the parents can have confidence in and trust. Birth is such an emotional time for both parents.

The woman is in a vulnerable position anyway and may act very sensitive at the end of the first stage of labor before she is fully dilated and expulsion begins. She may speak harshly to her husband and although he may understand why, he may brood. Or she may feel that he is acting optimistic to make her feel better because he loves her. But if the birth attendant says, "I can see a good deal of the head," the mother seems to believe her more.

Finally, the birth attendant is just a handy person to have around the house. If there is an older child who needs a glass of juice or if the doorbell rings or if another towel is needed, someone other than the husband should be able to meet these needs.

HOW TO CHOOSE A BIRTH ATTENDANT

But who should the birth attendant be? Without thinking a lot about it, most people would probably say they wanted a doctor, preferably an obstetrician, if one willing to come to the home could be found. One of the primary considerations of home birth is safety, and a doctor often appears to be the best insurance policy. He has had years of medical training and seems more experienced than any other kind of birth attendant you could find. He knows what to do in case of an emergency; he *could* even remove the baby surgically—though of course he wouldn't in the home; it is somehow reassuring that he knows how. (A midwife has not been schooled to do that.) The woman may also feel that her regular gynecologist knows her body best, from years of examining her.

But all this medical background may not really be an advantage in a home birth attendant. Actually, the only real advantage to having a doctor attend you at home is that, if by some chance you have to end up in the hospital for your baby's birth, your doctor can take you to the one he usually works in and deliver the baby there. If you were to show up yourself or with a midwife, you would probably become the new intern's learning experience for that day or the midwife wouldn't be allowed up with you or you might be treated in general as if you deserved to be prosecuted for endangering the life of your fetus.

Otherwise, there are several factors to consider before limiting your search for a home birth attendant to just doctors.

"Modern" Doctors

First and foremost, most doctors are male and white and have power and money. As such, they are members of the group which most oppresses women. Sometimes the oppression manifests itself in a condescending attitude toward the woman patient's intellectual and emotional capabilities. Doctors sometimes answer pregnant women's questions by telling their "pregnant gals" something like: "Don't, you worry your pretty little head about anything. Just follow my instructions, and I'll give you a healthy, happy baby."

Women doctors are sometimes better birth attendants than male doctors, but still they have been trained mostly by men in male-dominated medical schools and worked in male-dominated hospitals and other institutions. However, even if the woman doctor has never had a baby herself, she has probably at least been examined internally by a male doctor. Anyone who has ever stared between her thighs at a doctor's head as he putters around inside her while she lies flat on her back, feet in stirrups, has been subject to a humbling experience. And the quality of any birth attendant seems to rise in direct proportion to the amount of humility she or he is capable of.

A woman doctor is still a doctor, though, and the training of all doctors has been steeped in medicine, pathology, abnormality, surgery, and hospitals. With this background, it is hard for them to understand that the best thing a doctor can do at a home birth is to sit around in someone's bedroom for eight to twelve hours or so, fingers itching, and, provided no event out of the ordinary occurs, do virtually nothing. It does seem rather a waste of talent and time that years of expensive medical training should come to this, while in the outside world needy people suffer for lack of quality medical care.

Most doctors have never seen a normal, natural birth since attending home birth is no longer a requirement of medical school. So obstetricians rarely practice perineal massage or direct a slow delivery of the baby's head or encourage physiological birth positions, all of which nearly eliminate the need for episiotomy. What they have seen is routine episiotomy, and so this is what seems normal to them. The medical establishment is conservative and slow to change, and some practices, like routine episiotomy, have been repeated so often, though they may have been developed originally for medical emergencies, that social and cultural custom have made them seem part of the normal birth process. Some doctors do not realize that their own good intentions have led to overuse of some of the sophisticated techniques, which have caused other problems which are solved by using more techniques. Doctors are highly skilled to treat the *abnormal,* the medical problem, which birth usually is not.

Another factor which makes doctors unlikely candidates for home birth attendants is their ego. David Stewart of NAPSAC has commented, "I have learned the following advice for dealing with obstetricians: Don't tell an OB something he already knows. And don't tell an OB something he doesn't already know." The reverence afforded doctors in this country makes it hard for most of them to relinquish their godlike role and allow a woman to expel her own baby with the help of her husband and only minimal assitance from the doctor.

It should be remembered, of course, that individuals defy generalizations, and that some doctors make good home birth attendants. Certainly any doctor who is willing to do home birth exhibits less of the typical qualities than most other doctors. Nancy Mills, a California midwife, once said, "I've been to a lot of home births where doctors were present, and they seem to be 100 percent involved and concerned with getting the baby out. Even home birth doctors who have that consciousness of home birth seem to be wanting to get the baby out, but aren't in the place of caring much about the personal self-gratification that the woman gets out of it and the initial importance of that relationship with her child. They do tend to be trained to the extent that they look for problems. And when your consciousness and your fear put you in a place of looking for problems, I tend to think that maybe you get more problems. When you go looking for trouble you find it."

If you do want to choose a doctor as your home birth attendant, you may have better luck with a family practitioner. These physicians are more interested in the family as a unit and usually are more understanding of the reasons for wanting home birth than a specialist might be.

Many home birth midwives require that a woman be checked by a physician at least once during the pregnancy, not only to rule out major diseases, but also because this doctor will be the medical backup, and it is useful for doctor and patient to meet. If not already done, blood samples for laboratory analyses can be taken at this time.

And one more word about doctors. Most written guidelines for women interested in alternative birth methods will advise the woman to first "discuss it with your doctor." This is a fine thing to do, provided you have prepared yourself with the question, "Now what do I expect to happen when I bring it up?

Traditional Midwives

Throughout history, however, doctors have never been the traditional birth attendants. Midwives—usually women—were. The midwife was commonly a respected older woman who had borne children herself and who now helped other women do the same. The skills she possessed were probably learned from her mother, who had also been the village midwife and who had learned from her mother. These skills varied from culture to culture but always included a lot of common sense and perhaps some magical, mystical powers. Universally, the midwife was known as the comfort and support of the birthing woman.

As civilization developed, some midwives were burned as witches, and as medicine, science, and doctors grew in stature they increasingly discredited the art of midwifery when it was practiced by women midwives. The typical midwife was seen as unclean and unintelligent. Definitely she was un-degreed, and since only M.D.s could deliver babies in hospitals, when the trend toward hospitalized birth began in the 1900s the midwife was seen as unnecessary. Granny midwives, as nondegree midwives are sometimes known, existed in rural areas, and still do today, mainly in parts of the American South. But it is only through the recent home birth movement that their status in the community is being resurrected nationwide. These midwives are sometimes now called lay midwives, direct-entry midwives, or empirical midwives.

Modern Midwives

Another kind of midwife who exists in this country is the nurse-midwife. Some praise the development of the nurse-midwife during this century as the protection of women giving birth in hospitals, while others damn the development as organized medicine's trick to rid society forever of the granny midwife.

The history of the nurse-midwife goes back to 1917 when the United States Children's Bureau drew up a plan that included using nurses for full maternity care as a possible answer to the appallingly high infant mortality rate. A year later the Maternity Center Association was established in New York City. The founders felt the lack of maternity care training in nursing school was a glaring omission, and by 1931 they were setting up the first nurse-midwifery school in the country. At around the same time the Frontier Nursing Service (FNS) in Kentucky was going into full swing, showing how nurses could provide quality maternity care in the Appalachian backwoods, despite the relatively high risk factors of the childbearing population. In 1939 FNS opened its own college, and in 1944 the first university-affiliated nurse-midwives' school was opened.

Today, more than 50 years after formal nurse-midwifery education began, there are still not enough schools approved by the American College of Nurse-Midwives (ACNM), founded in 1955, to meet the number of applicants each year. And the schools, which offer either a certificate or master's degree in midwifery, are not graduating enough nurse-midwives to meet consumer demand. The ACNM refresher course had enabled some foreign-trained nurse-midwives to receive accreditation, but there are still fewer midwives in this country for its population than in almost every other civilized country in the world. Ina May Gaskin of The Farm notes, "We live in one of the only two countries in the world (the U.S. and Canada), as far as I can tell, that ever tried to abolish midwifery. The midwives did not organize in the early days while the doctors did."[3] Individual states and legal jurisdictions throughout the country make their own determinations about whether C.N.M.'s or lay midwives may obtain a license to practice in or out of a hospital.

The main source of opposition to licensing nurse-midwives to practice has been doctors. They have felt threatened by nurse-midwives, and for many years CNMs have not been permitted to deliver babies in hospitals, even though delivering babies is the purpose of their degree. They have merely to assist doctors, like any nonmidwife nurse. Finally, the increasing pressure of consumers, a shortage of doctors, and the need for those M.D.s who were in the field to be freed to concentrate their already limited time on medical complications forced in 1971 true recognition of CNMs. In that year a Joint Statement on Maternity Care from ACOG, the Nurses Association of ACOG and the ACNM proclaimed that "in medically directed teams, qualified nurse-midwives may assume responsibility for the complete care and management of uncomplicated maternity patients."[4] While there are still doctors who refuse to accept the nurse-midwife, others heap lavish praise, particularly since nondegree or lay midwives are again gaining status through the home birth movement. Certified nurse-midwives, at least, are establishment midwives, whose own accrediting agency, the ACNM, emphasizes that a nurse-midwife always functions with physician backup and may not be an independent practitioner. That may explain why for many years the hierarchy in nurse-midwifery opposed home birth. These older nurse-midwives had worked long and hard to gain recognition as a specialty in nursing, from other nurses, and in hospital obstetrics, from doctors.

At a grass-roots level, however, a new reality was evolving. Those handful of CNMs who were attending home births were more and more often crossing paths with a new breed of unlicensed midwife, usually called the lay midwife. Between the time the birth place swung to the hospital and most granny midwives retired, and the time the trend started swinging back but most doctors and nurse-midwives refused to come to the home, a gap developed. The modern lay midwife came into existence to fill that gap. Also nondegreed, modern lay midwives differ from traditional granny midwives in two main respects: their age and, for most, their desire to be an advocate of women's health care rights. Most lay midwives now have young families of their own, while traditional grannies were usually granny-age at the time they practiced their art.

What they do have in common with grannies is their fervent dedication. It is not uncommon for today's lay midwife to combine the time-consuming pressured existence of her profession with waking at dawn to care for her family, spending money on babysitters, transportation, and medical supplies (though she may receive little or no payment for her services), and then receive hateful looks from hospital emergency room nurses and doctors, although the mother and baby she brings with her may have remained alive because of the midwife's quick-thinking efforts.

The home birth movement has brought together many licensed CNMs and unlicensed midwives, who find there are many opportunities to learn from one another in the home setting. After all, they have the same interest at heart: to treat birth as a normal, healthy event that should enhance a family relationship. Also, since it always works to the advantage of the organization in power (in this case, the doctor-controlled medical establishment) if the oppressed are divided, both groups of midwives realized they had to stick together. Both were feeling the heat, whether they had been graduated from an ACNM-approved school or not. Thus, in 1982, Sr. Angela Murdagh, then president of the ACNM, brought together seven lay and certified midwives in a historic dialogue for modern midwives. These seven then went on to form MANA: the Midwives Alliance of North America. Hundreds of midwives are now members of the group, whose purpose is to increase communication among professional midwives of all backgrounds, as well as to ensure standards of care.

What all this means to you in choosing a birth attendant is that if you seek a nurse-midwife for your home birth, you will be choosing someone who, like a physician, has a medical/hospital background. Additionally she is someone who has been trained to function as part of a medical team, under an obstetrician's supervision, not as an independent—and having been a nurse first, she is further imbued with a subservient role in the medical hierarchy. But she will be in a situation, the home, where independent judgment is essential, and an obstetrician may be miles away. If, despite this medical background and almost certain ostracism by senior CNMs, she is still willing to attend you at home, you can be sure you have a person so dedicated to her art that she trained for her profession although, before 1971, she couldn't have been sure she would be allowed to practice it.

If you seek a lay midwife, however, it may be more difficult to determine her competency. Many lay midwives are skilled professionals, but a few who call themselves midwives are mothers who have set up shop after "helping out" at a few friends' births. Therefore, it is important for you to be able to determine your prospective midwife's level of training and experience. In the few states where lay midwifery is legal, there are excellent schools of midwifery, not under the control of the ACNM, that don't require a woman to be a nurse before admission. But if your midwife was taught more informally, how did she receive her education? (There are some groups that offer good home study courses, but then, what has been her supervised hands-on experience?) And if your midwife has been arrested or otherwise legally harassed, this is also important information for you to know. Although she probably did nothing to warrant an arrest, how will it affect her care of you during pregnancy and birth?

No matter what kind of midwife you choose, the result will usually be good, since birth is usually good, if not tampered with. Adequate prenatal care and screening can rule out almost every major complication of birth. But for the small risk remaining, it is smart to have a birth attendant on the lookout. In most cases, a competent midwife is the best choice.

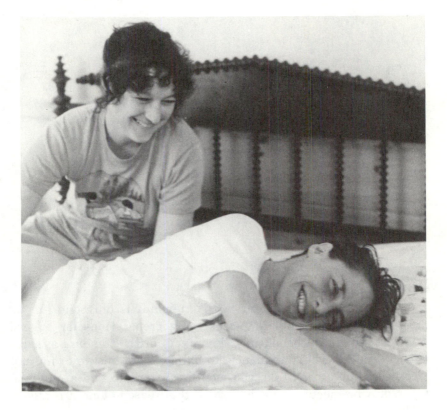

Byron Greatorex photograph

CHAPTER 6

Preparing for Birth

F inding a competent birth attendant is only one among many possibly time-consuming preparations for a good birth. It is beneficial to know your birth attendant as early as possible in your pregnancy, to build a relationship of mutual respect. But it may take you months of work to find a qualified person who meets your needs, so for that reason alone it is a good idea to start looking early.

FIND A BIRTH ATTENDANT

Even if there is a relatively well-known organized home birth service operating in your community, your regular doctor may not volunteer the information. So you will have to solicit leads on your own. Do ask the doctor anyway—not just an obstetrician, but a pediatrician and family practitioner too—and then put in calls to the medical society, health department, and hospitals in your area. Even if they say they know nothing about home birth attendants, it is good to let them know home birth is being requested. At hospitals, ask the director of nurse-midwifery, if there is one, as well as the directors of nursing and obstetrics. If you live in a relatively small town with a relatively small hospital, it may be possible to see these department heads after working hours, since sometimes what they won't tell you on the phone from their offices they will tell you in person. Individual doctors, residents and interns, nurse-midwives, and nurses may also help, if you manage to speak to them in person.

If midwifery is legal where you live, you can call the government agency which grants licenses to midwives and ask for a list of names. Your county clerk or department of health may know. In some jurisdictions being licensed or registered may just mean the person is "of sound mind and body" and paid the correct fee, but at least you have some leads. If midwifery is illegal, however, there is a chance that home birth practitioners are probably not open about their work. Then the names of midwives will have to be provided by personal recommendation. By asking around enough you are bound to meet someone who knows someone who is a friend of a friend, who has had a home birth.

Ask at a La Leche League meeting. This organization deals with breastfeeding, but sometimes someone in it has had a home birth. Check if your locality has a Childbirth Education Association (CEA). Ask a Lamaze, Bradley, or other childbirth education instructor. Ask at a health food store. If your local newspaper or television station has done a story on home birth, phone or write the reporter to ask for suggestions. Finally, a couple of the organizations listed in the appendix of this book have a master list of home birth attendants in most, if not all, states.

LEARN ABOUT PREGNANCY AND BIRTH

The early part of your pregnancy is also the time to begin the process of self-education about birth, child care, and parenting. The more self-education a woman undertakes during her pregnancy the more positive she is likely to feel about the state of being pregnant and her upcoming birth and motherhood experiences. Knowledge is the key to feeling in control. Reading books, attending courses, and initiating discussions with new parents and childbirth educators may yield some conflicting information and challenge your ideas on home birth and mothering. But even if the only use you will make of the negative responses is to better prepare you for dealing with the reactions of those around you, the total exposure will be well worth it.

NUTRITION

Another early and important preparation for a good pregnancy and birth—even before conception, if possible—is to become an expert on nutrition. Good nutrition during pregnancy is probably the single most important factor in giving birth to a healthy baby. Home birth physician Mayer Eisenstein of Chicago once said that if he was forced to make a choice, he would choose a baby of a well-nourished mother who had been drugged for delivery over the baby of a "natural childbirth" mother who was poorly nourished during pregnancy.[1] But unfortunately, correct nutrition is rarely given its rightful place in any program of prenatal care. Prenatal care is not as good as it should be in this country because doctors feel they can cope with any emergency in the hospital. So if you are having a home birth it is especially important for you to take on the responsibility for good prenatal care yourself.

You will find that in general midwives appreciate the importance of good nutrition in pregnancy. Applied nutrition is rarely covered in medical school, and for too long doctors have not cared at all what the pregnant patient ate. If they recommended any diet, it was too sparse. Doctors asked women to keep their weight gain down to what we now see were dangerous levels; it was as if they were more interested in what her figure would be like at the six-week postpartum checkup than in the health of the baby. And there are still a lot of doctors who act this way. It is important for you not to succumb to this kind of pressure, living as we do in a society which stresses that you can never be too thin. Keep remembering that a direct result of good nutrition is the near elimination of the chance of prematurity and low birthweight babies, as well as toxemia. This has been shown over and over by people like obstetrician Tom Brewer and dietitian Agnes Higgins of Canada, among others.[2] Other studies have linked prematurity and low birthweight to cerebral palsy, mental retardation, and other brain disorders.

Recent research shows us that good nutrition during pregnancy affects the child even years later. In 1981 an international team of investigators reported that even mild caloric deficiencies in the diet of an infant or pregnant woman can disturb a youngster's emotional stability as late as age six or eight. And in 1985 the journal *Pediatrics* reported on research showing visual-motor co-ordination difficulties in school children who had been very low birthweight newborns. Accompanying diagrams from the actual research study showed the faltering pencilled attempts of five year olds who couldn't copy a triangle or an asterisk when their normal birthweight counterparts could.[3]

And, according to the National Academy of Sciences, babies weighing less than 5.5 lb. at birth are almost forty times more likely to die during their first month of life than babies above that weight. While for years doctors taught that the fetus was "like a parasite"—it would take from the mother what it needed no matter what she ate—we now know this is not true. Even so, in 1986 the National Center for Health Statistics (NCHS) reported that 23 percent of American mothers gained less than 16 lb. during pregnancy.[4] While stating that women with a higher education generally had a reduced risk of low birthweight, the same report found that of the women who gained less than 16 lb. during pregnancy, there was no significant difference in the risk of low birthweight between those with less than a high school education and those who completed college. The NCHS report also said that the risk of fetal death decreased with additional weight gain; fetal death dropped nearly 50 percent as weight gain increased from less than 16 lb. to 26–35 lb.

In spite of all this knowledge and recent research, the food for babies issue has become part of the politics of federal spending. In 1986 the United States Department of Agriculture tried to obscure the positive results of a five-year study on its Women, Infants and Children (WIC) nutrition program by omitting or rewriting the data summaries. The study had credited the WIC program with reducing premature births and infant mortality, increasing birth-weights, and heightening the intellectual development of pres-choolers; but funding for this program has been frozen since 1981. It is no wonder that the Childrens Defense Fund has found the infant mortality rate rising a few percent per year![5]

This research only serves to emphasize that pregnant women cannot underestimate the importance of nutrition. Great emphasis must be placed not only on *enough* weight gain but enough protein, since this is the stuff of which life is made. You should aim for a protein intake of 100 grams per day. The usual plentiful source of potein is meat, including poultry and fish. Meat also is a good source of iron. But beef and poultry may have fillers which can be dangerous, fish may contain chemicals like PCBs, and all three are usually expensive. So other sources of protein may be used. These include milk, cheese, and eggs and also soybeans, nuts, and lentils. Remember that a quart of milk and two eggs contain about 40 grams right there. The protein intake should be supplemented by plenty of fresh fruits and vegetables and whole grains. Vegetarians also can have healthy pregnancy diets if they are careful to eat foods in the right combinations to satisfy the required protein intake. Lacto-ovo vegetarians should take a vitamin B_{12} supplement.

Avoid Pollutants

Food contaminants must be considered because they do pass through the placenta, and side-effects to the developing fetus are being discovered. There is no food which is totally free from environmental pollutants. Nitrites in luncheon meat and frankfurters are carcinogenic and reduce oxygen in the blood; monosodium glutamate has been shown to cause genetic changes. Shopping in a supermarket, which most of us do, makes it impossible to avoid contaminated foods. Fruits are sprayed with insecticide, and most vegetables grow in soil filled with unnatural chemicals. Milk is good for us, but cows eat grass covered with strontium 90. And on and on. Even unsprayed produce may be covered with insecticde that drifted over from the farm five miles away. Even most health food stores have some products with additives, or "natural" products which may be covered by a potentially dangerous plastic wrapping. According to the Food and Drug Administration (FDA), about 3,000 substances are intentionally added to foods to produce a desired effect. As many as 10,000 other compounds or combinations of compounds find their way into various foods during processing, packaging, or storage. The FDA cites as examples infinitesimal residues of pesticides used to treat crops, minute amounts of drugs fed to animals, and chemical substances that migrate from plastic packaging materials. Indeed, sometimes it seems as if there is no way to eat healthy foods.

The goal, then, is to minimize additives by eating foods in as close to their natural state as possible. Everyone's eating habits can be improved in some way. If you are drinking soda with meals, replace it with juice. If you're buying canned vegetables, try frozen. If you're buying frozen, try fresh. If you're boiling vegetables, learn to steam them. Or just throw them raw into a salad. Foods should be cooked enough to destroy germs, not vitamins, so don't overcook. Try to eat as little processed and refined food as possible. Stop eating mushy white bread. If you can't replace it all with whole wheat bread, make your sandwiches with one slice of each. Try to eliminate white sugar from your diet or at least keep it to a minimum. When having guests, serve raisins and nuts or cheese, not candy. Chemical sweeteners are also harmful, and so is a lot of coffee. On the positive side, supplement your diet healthfully by sprinkling in a couple of tablespoons of brewer's yeast when making spaghetti sauce or adding wheat germ to recipes when you would ordinarily use just bread crumbs. To protect yourself against food side-effects yet to be discovered, another good ground rule is not to eat an excess of any one kind of food over a period of time.

Besides the caffeine in coffee (and in colas, tea, and chocolate), which miscellaneous reports have linked with increasing rates of spontaneous abortion and birth defects, there are a number of other drugs that pregnant women should avoid. Recently, the most highly publicized of these is alcohol, because of new research on increased drinking rates of women of childbearing age. The effects of light or moderate drinking on the fetus are not well documented, but the effects of 4–5 oz. of 100-proof alcohol per day can cause fetal alcohol syndrome, characterized by severe growth deficiency, heart defects, malformed facial features, and mental retardation. Only 1 oz. of alcohol stops fetal growth for one hour, preventing the growth of fifteen million brain cells.

A related concern is smoking. The effects of smoking on the fetus are so well documented now that the federal government was able to override the powerful tobacco lobby and require warnings on packages of cigarettes. Cigarette smoke contains over one thousand drugs. Only a few of them—such as nicotine, carbon monoxide, cyanide, and DDT—have been tested for effects on the fetus, and they are all harmful. This means that even if you don't smoke, you must be especially vigilant about second-hand smoke reaching you and your baby, from cigarettes smoked by others at your place of work or among your family. Since recent research has shown that in some ways second-hand smoke is more harmful than inhaled smoke, you may have to raise a protest or change your seat at work and ask otherwise thoughtful relatives not to smoke in your presence. You certainly have the right to forbid smoking in your own home.

As for other drugs ingested during pregnancy, they are too numerous to review for all their side-effects. It is wise to remember that most every drug taken by a pregnant woman reaches the fetus, and this includes over-the-counter remedies. In one published study, 97 percent of women took prescribed drugs and 65 percent took self-administered drugs. Recent research has shown that aspirin used within several weeks of birth is linked with interference in the neonatal clotting mechanism and jaundice. Another type of drug commonly prescribed for women, tranquilizers such as *Valium* and *Librium* and others containing meprobamate or benzodiazepine, have been shown to increase the risk of cleft lip or palate. Although more study is needed to determine the effects on the unborn baby of "street drugs," according to the March of Dimes, there is no question that they imperil the woman's health, and that increases the user's chance of having a sick baby. In addition, drugs used to combat nausea and vomiting in pregnancy have recently been found to be harmful. If you are nauseous in pregnancy, reconsider your diet. Small amounts of high protein and complex carbohydrates eaten as snacks throughout the day and the other principles of good nutrition discussed, are the main non-drug ways to treat nausea in pregnancy.

With the kind of diet that stresses a protein intake of 100 grams per day, plus a lot of fruits, vegetables, and whole grains, you will probably gain at least 30 lb. during pregnancy. This is good. Even a weight gain of 50 or 60 lb. should not be cause for despair, especially if you were thin before pregnancy. As long as the quality of the gain is high, the number of pounds should not be considered important. Yet weight gain in pregnancy is one area where pregnant women may be in conflict with their doctors, due to antiquated belief systems.

Another area of conflict has been the use of salt during pregnancy. Salt is a necessary nutrient, not only because all cells are bathed in saline solution, but because salt in pregnancy supports the 40 to 60 percent increase in blood volume which is necessary to service the placenta and baby. This increased fluid volume also helps protect against shock after the normal loss of fluids after birth, and prepares the body for breastfeeding. Therefore, swelling during pregnancy is a normal symptom for a well-nourished woman, as long as her blood pressure is normal, and should be relieved simply by elevating the feet. The mother should not cut down on her salt, and in no case should she take diuretics.[6]

Vitamins and minerals are routinely prescribed during pregnancy, although some of the common brands have BHA and BHT as preservatives. Most doctors give away samples that the drug company salesperson left at the last visit. Doctors may criticize the woman if she refuses to take them. Some women prefer to analyze their own individual diets and then take only those supplements they feel are necessary, for example, folic acid or iron. Remember, supplements are just that and cannot substitute for real food. Additionally, some babies are affected by overdoses of common vitamins. Vitamin A over 18,000 I.U. per day can cause fetal cataracts, bone fragility, and enlarged spleen and liver, and Vitamin D overdose prevents fetal weight gain and can lead to kidney damage.

AMNIOCENTESIS, AND OTHER INTERVENTIONS

Other hazards of pregnancy, to which more and more women are exposing themselves, are amniocentesis and other, experimental tests that attempt to detect abnormalities in the fetus. In amniocentesis, a needle is inserted into the uterus for the purpose of withdrawing amniotic fluid for analysis. The test is done in the fourth month of pregnancy. A sonogram should precede the needle insertion so the fetus itself or the placenta is not stabbed. The fluid contains cells sloughed off the baby and can be analyzed for certain abnormalities, such as Down's syndrome. It takes at least two weeks to obtain results. Since the chance of having a Down's syndrome baby increases with age and since women are having babies at later ages, almost all doctors encourage or try to require women, even those below the age of thirty-five, to have amniocentesis. This pressure is applied even to women who state they would not have an abortion, especially an advanced pregnancy abortion, even if the baby had Down's syndrome.

Women who want amniocentesis should have full disclosure on the potential risk first and then weigh the risk-benefit ratio. One vigorously controlled study conducted by the Medical Research Council Working Party on Amniocentesis in England compared

2,428 women who had amniocentesis with 2,428 matched controls who did not, in nine British obstetrics centers. The children born were followed up until the age of ten months. The results showed that in the amniocentesis group, there were clearly apparent an excess risk of spontaneous abortion (miscarriage), an excess risk of serious hemorrhage related to an increase in both abruption and placenta previa, an excess risk of the infant's having unexplained respiratory difficulties at birth lasting for more than twenty-four hours, a similar excess of major orthopedic postural deformities, and an increased risk of Rh contamination. Overall, perinatal mortality was twenty in the amniocentesis group and eleven in the controls.[7]

A more recent study, which appeared in *Ob/Gyn News* (1986), concludes that amniocentesis causes miscarriage in about one in every 200 procedures. Also, doctors have found that approximately 5 percent of infants who had amniocentesis show dimplelike needle marks on their bodies as they grow. These needle marks, which apparently were not noticed at birth but became visible as the skin grew and stretched, indicate that more babies are touched by the needles than was previously believed.

There are two even newer tests, still in the experimental stage, which pregnant women are coming under increasing pressure to accept. In California, physicians are required by law to offer one of the tests, the alpha fetoprotein (AFP) blood test, to their patients. In this test, the level of alpha fetoprotein excreted by the fetus into the mother's bloodstream is measured. Large amounts of AFP may be caused by a neural tube defect, either anencephaly or spina bifida. In 1984 it was discovered that low amounts of AFP may indicate a chromosomal defect such as Down's syndrome. The blood test is given at about sixteen weeks of pregnancy, and suspicious levels are followed up by sonogram and amniocentesis.

An even more controversial test is chorionic villi sampling (CVS). This test is performed in the first trimester, when there can be a so-called "easier" abortion, and the results are available faster than with amniocentesis. For CVS, the cells for analysis are removed from the villi on the chorion, which surrounds the fetus in early pregnancy. When the test was first introduced in this country in 1983, an FDA-regulated plastic catheter for removing the cells was inserted through the cervix up to the chorion. But nowadays many obstetricians use a needle through the abdomen, an unregulated technique since the FDA doesn't regulate techniques, only devices and drugs. Also, on the chorionic villi tissue, there is more of a chance that maternal and fetal cells could mix, yielding incorrect results.

Since there are now three such tests where pregnant women are encouraged to "deal with" less than perfect fetuses, with the implication that all should be aborted, we must continue to question the direction in which we are heading. Do we get rid of a loving child with Down syndrome because she is slow to learn and keep the so-called normal person because he has the ability to think of these tests?

PHYSICAL WELL-BEING

Another possible hazard during pregnancy is car accidents, the number one cause of nonobstetric deaths of pregnant women in the U.S. Although seat belt injuries have occurred to the fetus when pregnant women were involved in accidents, a study showed that the risk of death to both mother and baby is far greater if pregnant women do not use seat belts. The researchers concluded that failure to wear seat belts far outweighs the risk to the fetus from the seat belt itself.[8]

Another important part of maintaining prenatal health is exercise. Some exercise programs for pregnancy developed by well-known celebrities and their associates have spurred the American College of Obstetricians & Gynecologists to develop guidelines and issue its videotape for commercial distribution. While the ACOG video is admittedly more conservative than the more popular ones, all the exercise promoters agree on certain principles. One is that exercise during pregnancy does help a pregnant woman with the stress and strain of pregnancy. Another is that women who are very active prior to pregnancy probably can continue that level of activity well into the pregnancy, and women who are not as active are generally safe in attempting moderate exercise.

Of course, you do not need to purchase an exercise video to stay in shape during pregnancy. Walking a mile a day, plus one other exercise like swimming or stationary cycling, are probably all that are needed. If you take a "pregnercise" course at your local "Y," be sure not to do any exercising on your back, because the weight of the baby and uterus on the vena cava, which carries blood back to the heart, can cause compression, reducing the heart's output of oxygen-rich blood to the fetus. (This also applies to sleeping on your back during pregnancy.)

Posture, though not exercise in the popular sense, is an important consideration for pregnancy. As the baby grows, the center of gravity changes, and some women compensate by arching in their lower back and "waddling like a duck," increasing the chance of developing lower back problems, a common complaint of pregnancy. Instead, the stomach muscles should be held pressed against the baby, with the pelvis tilted back by tucking under the buttocks. Doing a "pelvic rock" on hands and knees also helps. Pregnant women should also learn Kegel exercises which strengthen the pubococcygeal muscle. The recent television advertising of products for older women with bladder control problems highlights the importance of building up the muscles that support the contents of a woman's pelvis, especially during pregnancy when those contents weigh much more, and during childbirth, when those muscles are stretched to capacity.

PREPARED CHILDBIRTH EDUCATION

Reading books on birth, even before pregnancy if possible, will help you determine which type of childbirth education course you wish to attend. In some localities there is choice, but in others there is none. In general, the Lamaze method has a stronghold on the eastern half of the United States, and the Bradley method is better known in the West. There are also other childbirth methods, such as those developed by Dick-Read and Sheila Kitzinger, which may appeal to you. Even if there is little choice of classes in your area, the books you read will help you adapt what you learn in classes to meet your desires. The instructors in some classes teach what amounts to a combination of methods, so after reading books by and about Dick-Read, Kitzinger, Lamaze, Bradley, and possibly others, it is a good idea to talk to the instructor before registering for the course.

Dr. Grantly Dick-Read was the first promoter of childbirth education to receive widespread attention among those interested in natural childbirth. His main and lasting contribution to childbirth education is his observation that fear of the unknown (childbirth) leads to tension, which leads to pain. Thus the Dick-Read method, like all childbirth education methods, begins with a discussion of the physiology of birth.

Sheila Kitzinger is another childbirth educator whose work is of interest. She is a popular lecturer when she visits the United States from England, where she does work for the famed National Childbirth Trust. Kitzinger's book, *The Experience of Childbirth,* is illustrated with photos of the birth of her twins at home, and she is the author of several other excellent books on birth. An anthropologist by schooling, Kitzinger calls her system of childbirth the psychosexual method. It is psychosexual because she attempts to integrate the childbirth experience with other aspects of a woman's sexuality. Kitzinger also understands a woman's body and feelings and uses excellent imagery to encourage a woman to teach herself how to relax different parts of her body. Kitzinger speaks of "greeting" each contraction.

The most popular promotor of childbirth preparation was probably Dr. Fernand Lamaze, a French obstetrician who toured Russian birth clinics and "discovered" that Pavlovian stimulus-and-response methods were being used by laboring women. He brought this conditioned response method of distraction and panting patterns back to Paris, where his clinic still stands; the method was popularized in the United States by Marjorie Karmel, an American patient of Dr. Lamaze who returned to New York and wrote the engaging, *Thank You, Dr. Lamaze.* In 1960 she teamed with Elisabeth Bing, a registered physical therapist from Europe, to begin the American Society for Psychoprophylaxis in Obstetrics (ASPO), the group which trains and certifies Lamaze teachers. Marjorie Karmel has since died, but Elisabeth Bing has gone on to become a prolific author and holder of an appointment at a prestigious New York medical college, uplifting the status of childbirth education in this country. Both Elisabeth Bing and ASPO headquarters have remained on the East Coast, contributing to that method's predominance in that part of the country.

On the West Coast, the Bradley method is more popular. Dr. Robert Bradley is a Denver obstetrician who pioneered the concept of fathers in the delivery room as the mother's chief "coach." His method stresses nutrition, consumer awareness, and using progressive relaxation with deep, slow, sleeplike breathing during labor, not panting. An even newer method that is similar to the Bradley method is Cooperative Childbirth, developed by Gail Brewer, a well-known author and childbirth educator, and promoted by Childbirth Education Association's Metropolitan New

York chapter, which Brewer co-founded. Cooperative Childbirth means the woman learns to cooperate with her body, and everyone else learns to cooperate with the woman. These last two methods are considered an improvement on Lamaze, whose method has been criticized for causing hyperventilation and tension, especially in connection with forceful pushing, and for being too doctor-controlled. Many women prefer systems which are more physiological and teach a woman to ride with her contractions rather than distract herself from them.

Home birth parents will be more comfortable in classes where the teacher stresses consumer control and choices, not unquestioning cooperation with the hospital procedure. A good childbirth class should include a healthy questioning attitude on the part of parents and a healthy dose of discussions on options available. Sometimes asking to see a prospective childbirth teacher's handouts will give you an idea of the type of attitude that is fostered. Parents preparing for a vaginal birth after a previous cesarean should look for special VBAC preparation classes because they will answer the special needs of this group—anger over their cesarean and positive visualization of a normal birth this time.

There is always the woman who can have a satisfying labor and birth without any prior training or education, if a midwife or labor coach can help her along with slow deep breathing and relaxation during contractions. But taking a course is recommended because there is always something to be learned. Many women and men find that being with other expectant couples helps the baby's father verbalize his feelings, feel less excluded from birth and more accepting of his important role. Good childbirth educators know how to adapt their lessons for women without partners, adolescents, or people who may be distrusting. A childbirth teacher in your area who is known to be a patients' advocate in her work would probably be the kind most willing to adapt her methods or offer special suggestions for birth at home. Some lay midwives started out as childbirth instructors, so see if your childbirth attendant herself runs classes.

EDUCATE YOUR FAMILY AND FRIENDS

Pregnancy is also the time to prepare those close to you for the birth. How soon you tell well-meaning but nervous friends and relatives, such as the grandparents-to-be, that you are planning to have the baby at home varies with the individual relationships.

It is helpful to share thoughts and books with loved ones but try not to be disappointed at not receiving total support from them.

If you have a child or children under the age of about twelve living in your house at the time of birth, you may want to choose one or two adults and ask them to attend your birth specifically for the purpose of caring for the child or children. These adults should be respectful of your reasons for home birth, since negative vibrations are not helpful while you labor and give birth. These adults should be well prepared for what birth at home will be like. Pass on to them books you are reading and initiate discussions so they can have their questions answered. Your children should feel close to these people, too, because while you and your husband are concentrating on the birth, your child may need another person for company. These adults must be willing to be on call and leave their jobs or disturb their sleep whenever you contact them. Beforehand they need to understand what will be expected of them that day, such as being there in case your child wakes up or preparing meals and dressing, bathing, and playing with the child if necessary. If your child is disruptive—which she or he probably won't be if also prepared by you—the close friends or relatives may have to take her or him outside, though they may want to attend the birth themselves. Some couples with older children have happy home births without other adults present and are able to cope with the needs of their children as well. But it will probably be helpful for all of you if you can find another relative or close friend to be there as well.

There must be good rapport with these adults or any others you invite to your birth. If many people are planning to attend the celebration, it may be a good idea to tell your midwife. It is possible, and perhaps your friends should be told this, too, that if the birth attendant feels your labor is slowing down or you aren't relaxed or certain individuals create noticeable tension, she may ask them to leave the room. Although many people may be your friends, those you invite to the birth have to be people with whom you feel comfortable opening up.

If you do have older children, their preparation should be more extensive, depending on the age of each child. In general, you should tell children as much as they are capable of understanding (usually more than we think). With children, too, knowledge alleviates fear.

The sooner you start, the better. Even a two-year-old child is capable of understanding, "Mommy's going to the doctor today for a checkup," and then a simple statement why. Matter-of-factly telling your older child what is happening each step of the way will help her or him to accept the birth as fact. Share pictures of births in books with your child; describe what sounds or faces you may make if you have to push; ask your child to imagine what it would feel like to have a baby coming through; and assure your child that she or he came out of your body that way as well. Of course, discussions should be made reassuringly, with allowance for questions and time for closeness and special attention afterward. Children should be informed that some blood comes out when the baby is born, but that is okay. A mature child of four or five or older might be told that if there is too much bleeding or if the baby acts sick right after birth, you both might have to go to the hospital for extra help. But this doesn't have to be stressed, as it is very unlikely to happen.

Many parents, those planning hospital births included, think that a sibling need not be told about the new baby until shortly before the birth. These parents may not realize that the child notices the changes in the mother's body or hears her talk about the "new baby" or "the doctor." If the tone of voice is secretive, an older child may imagine that something much less pleasant than a new baby is about to happen.

Some mothers may also feel that sharing a lot of talk about the new baby may make the older child jealous. But if discussion is done on a gradual basis, as things cross your mind as part of the daily routine, the older child slowly accepts the new baby as part of her or his future reality, the same way you and your partner do. It is also important to note that if there is to be jealousy, most of it will manifest itself after the baby is born. But, since you will not be separated by hospitalization from your older child, which many psychologists feel is the start of such resentment, you may find, as some home birth mothers do, that the older child is not jealous at all. Lee Stewart of NAPSAC has said, "If a child is allowed to be involved in the birth of his brother or sister and actually see the baby emerge from the mother, we feel that the child will realize that the baby is physically a part of the mother and will have no trouble accepting the baby just as he has already accepted his mother."

Whether older children should view the actual birth is a big concern to some parents, as well as to many relatives and acquaintances. This is something you must decide on yourself, because if the birthing mother is not comfortable about who is in the birth room with her she may not enjoy the birth and she may actually hold back on its progress. You should know that many home birth parents have noticed that letting the sibling see the baby being born opens up the opportunity for a close relationship between the children from the start. One day more scientific study will be done on the bonding between newborns and siblings at a home birth. At present, we are only just beginning to understand the complexities of mother-infant bonding.

Many parents feel that the best way to decide whether the older children view the birth is to see what happens at the time. If a child is awake and not disrupting the work of the parents and the birth attendant and responds well to the person invited to care for the child, there is no reason to make a point of excluding him. Most older children just drift in and out of the room, and if they see birth is near, they stay—or there is a possibility they may not even notice or care. If a very young child is asleep, it is usually just as well to let her sleep, since the child may awaken cranky and confused. You might want to have a discussion with any child of about three or older during your ninth month of pregnancy to see how she feels about being awakened or called home from school.

Other people worry over whether a mother should let her child see her wide-open vagina and whether the child will be upset by the blood and noises which accompany birth. As for seeing a vagina, most parents contemplating home birth seem to be the kind of people who have let their children see them naked and have given information on the body's sex organs, so this usually is not an issue—except in other people's minds. As for the blood of childbirth, you will see that children are beautifully accepting of birth and what accompanies it, if they have been prepared for what to expect and if the adults in the room, especially the birth attendant, are acting confidently. A mature child may even make a good labor coach or may have a specific job, such as wetting the washcloth or minding the tape recorder.

Probably the worst mistake you could make, regarding older children in your birth room, is to forcibly exclude the child, under protest, such as by locking the door or just refusing to let him in. Then the child may become hysterical, wanting to see his mother, and with the help of imagination, harmfully misinterpret words, noises, and glimpses. It is also not advantageous to pack away your child from the house for a week when you begin labor, as one birth book advises, since all the advantages of home birth to the siblings are negated, and the children have to cope additionally with the absence of their parents and their belongings.

RELATIONS WITH YOUR PARTNER

Your older child isn't the only person who requires special conversations or preparation. Your husband is another. Especially if this is your first pregnancy your husband also is probably going through many changes. Some of these changes, like yours, may be physical. Some husbands actually gain weight or experience more aches and discomfort during their wives' pregnancies. More commonly, their concerns are in their minds. Your mate may wonder if he will be a good father, if he will make enough money, how he will share the child care, if he will lose some of his freedom or some of your affection, if he can hurt the baby when you have sex, if he feels as positive as you about wanting a home birth, and what he should do if the birth attendant doesn't arrive on time. You will want to share your books and thoughts with your husband and encourage discussions of these topics, especially if he is not usually the type to verbalize his thoughts and emotions.

One area of concern to both parents deserves mention here, and that is sex during pregnancy. A woman may think that pregnancy makes her less attractive. She may feel uncomfortable in what she considers the "man's" sex position. A man may fear that intercourse will hurt the baby. For whatever reasons, many couples find that pregnancy changes their sex habits in ways that are not enjoyable or necessary, particularly if this adds up to months of abstention. Sometimes the problem is lack of communication between the couple on how each feels about sex during pregnancy. More often the problem has been the reticence of the medical profession. Most doctors offer little advice about sex during pregnancy except to recommend that it be halted six weeks before the due date. In truth, with few exceptions, there need be no abstinence at all during pregnancy. There is some evidence to suggest that women with a history of miscarriage may do better to avoid deep penile penetration or orgasm until the fourth month of pregnancy. Of course, after a woman's bag of waters breaks at the beginning or during labor, she should avoid intercourse or she is increasing the risk of infection. Bleeding and pain at the end of pregnancy would also be contraindications for having sex, probably because it would mean the prostaglandins in the semen were irritating the ripe cervix. But on the whole, women with normal pregnancies should feel free to have intercourse as often as they like throughout the end of pregnancy. A woman's orgasm by itself is not responsible for premature labor. The only sexual practice the medical literature shows is surely risky during pregnancy is blowing air into the vagina. A few cases of fatal air emboli have been reported.

You and your partner will probably want to discuss your feelings and try new positions and practices. It is normal if, during your pregnancy, you experience some loss of interest in sex, and it is also normal if, at other times, such as around your fourth month when the blood vessels in your belly begin to enlarge, you find you are more sensitive and stimulated about sex. It is important to remember that all pregnancy-based difficulties with sex are temporary, and that it is especially important now, as in all good and bad crises in a relationship, to communicate. There are many ways of expressing love, and changing your attitude may lead to new and creative methods of lovemaking. If you are having difficulties, start with learning massage techniques on each other, reminding your partner of the importance of massage for relaxation during labor. Practice your techniques on each other while naked, using oil on your hands to reduce friction. Many couples find it is easier to be spontaneous during pregnancy because it is the only time they don't have to worry about getting pregnant.

But the one person going through the most changes, who needs the most time and special attention, is you. It is your body, your baby, your pregnancy. Everything about these nine months really belongs to you.

Pregnancy has been described as an altered state of consciousness by Arthur and Libby Colman, whose research deals with the psychological aspects of pregnancy. They show that emotional vulnerability is a characteristic of pregnancy and that it is caused not only by hormonal changes but also by such factors as feelings about and experience with independence and dependence, separateness and growth, even memories of our own fetal existence.[9] Feelings of losing freedom and identity are not uncommon. We fought so long to be known as teacher, writer, lawyer, welder, secretary, not just "wife"; now with what status will the identity of "mother" place us? It is important for you to arrive at the realization that you are still you, that your new title will be just another enriching aspect of you. At best, you have resolved most of your conflicts about freedom and identity regarding your work and play outside the home before becoming pregnant. Pregnancy and motherhood are times to reorder priorities.

Some women also worry about whether they will be adequate mothers, and it is good to know that there are a lot of places where a woman can share her feelings on the subject. La Leche League meetings are a good place to go to meet other pregnant women like yourself who are interested in getting their children off to a good start in life. The fact that you are having a home birth shows that your are the kind of parent who is willing to accept the responsibility of parenthood and make intelligent decisions you feel are in the best interests of your child and family.

All parents, not only those planning home birth, worry about the possibility of giving birth to a malformed or sick baby. Such thoughts and bad dreams about them are normal, and you should not fear them as premonitions. You realize that the possibility of your having a baby born with a problem has been greatly reduced by your good diet and the planned lack of unnecessary intervention into the normal processes. If your child is born with a problem, you will be better able to accept it if you are conscious and with loved ones. Mothers who were unconscious during the birth of a baby with a cleft palate or worse have said they had a harder time accepting the problem.

WHAT YOU WILL NEED FOR THE BIRTH

The final area for preparation during your home birth pregnancy is your home. There are certain things you can do beforehand if you are the kind who likes to plan ahead to insure everything will go smoothly. But since most things like changing linens can be done by a helper while you're in labor, you don't have to be overly concerned about preparing your home. Probably your birth attendant will bring most of the things she needs and can make do with whatever else you have around the house. Most people have a large pot in their house for sterilizing scissors without being told that they should set one aside. But for those who can't always locate such things on short notice, here are some suggestions.

- You may want to use an old shower curtain as a plastic covering for your bed. Some couples put clean linens under the plastic so the bed is already made up for after the birth. They cover the plastic with an old sheet. This sheet will probably get blood and fluids on it so later you may want just to throw it out instead of washing it. If you do want to keep the top sheet, you may want to buy some disposable bed pads at a drugstore.
- You can also set aside the famous pot for boiling instruments and a pot or bowl to put the placenta in.
- Have a plastic trash bag ready to dispose of bloody things such as the placenta, bed pads, or sheet.
- Ask your birth attendant if you should have on hand any particular kind of large gauze pads, washcloths, or towels.
- Check if she is the one providing the bulb syringe, for possible suctioning of the baby's mucus, and the clamps and scissors for cutting the umbilical cord.
- You may also want to set aside after-birth outfits, not just for the baby but for yourself too. Remember, you will have to be able to nurse the baby in your outfit. Skin-to-skin contact is a good reason for both you and the baby to be naked after birth, but there should be covers over both of you so the baby doesn't lose body temperature if the room is not very warm.
- You will need sanitary pads, and the baby will need diapers.
- You may wish to ready an outfit to labor and give birth in, keeping in mind that by the time birth is near you may be most comfortable with nothing on at all. A birth outfit should be loose fitting, able to be lifted up from the bottom, for birth, and pulled down from the top, for breastfeeding. A robe which opens in front allows for both of these accesses, as well as for resting the baby on your bare skin. A robe can also be pulled around you if you are sitting and chatting with family and friends during early labor, wrapped tightly around you if you get chills in late labor, and quickly thrown open if the labor has made you hot and sticky.

One essential deserving advance planning in the home is food. It's a good idea to keep food and drink in stock so an important person doesn't have to go out looking for an open store if you labor and give birth at night. Keep plenty of frozen orange juice for energy. Keep plenty of frozen and canned foods for the birthday celebration in case there is no time or place to get fresh food. Buy more than enough for all who'll attend, because if your labor is long, people may be eating more than one full meal at your home. The food should be easy for anyone to serve, so that you and your mate don't have to concern yourselves with it. It is also a good idea, if you have the space, to freeze casserole-style dishes for quick serving after the baby is born. You will appreciate the advance preparation.

If you have an older child or children, it may be nice to include them in the planning of a birthday party. Let them buy small gifts to give the new baby, and you buy a few more for the baby to give them. And don't forget the champagne!

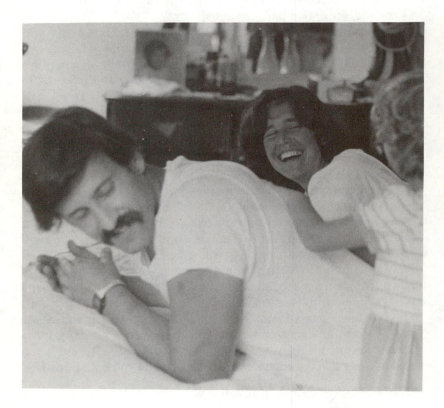

Byron Greatorex photograph

CHAPTER 7

Birth

I n the ninth month of pregnancy it is difficult to have perspective, to imagine what it was like when you were not pregnant. It is common to feel as if you have been pregnant forever. Sometimes it is hard to stand or walk for long periods of time. You may have trouble finding a comfortable position in which to sleep and may be waking up more than once during the night just to go to the bathroom. The weight of your uterus presses on your bladder, and it just doesn't hold as much as it used to. You are getting anxious. One mother, expecting twins, said, "I just want to meet them already."

Often at the end of a day when you are feeling your most lethargic, coming-down-with-a-cold-or-something, impatient and draggiest, labor begins. At its start labor may be distinguishable only to those who have experienced it before or those truly in tune with the rhythms of their bodies. Most of the rest of us, busy with activity at an office or school or home with children, recognize the start of labor only when more noticeable signs present themselves.

SIGNS OF LABOR

The earliest of these signs may be "bloody show." The mucus plug which caps the bottom part of the uterus (the cervix) breaks open and some mucus mixed with blood comes out through the vagina. Bloody show may be noticed on sheets or panties or on toilet paper after urinating. The appearance of bloody show means that labor is not far off. Contractions will probably start within a few days. Often contractions start that day.

Another indication that labor is starting is the spontaneous rupture of the membranes, usually referred to as the "breaking of the bag of waters"; the amniotic fluid that surrounds the baby in the uterus begins to leave the woman's body through her vagina. The fluid may come in a steady trickle, in spurts, or in a big gush. It is clear or whitish, distinguished from urine by smell and by the fact that you can't control it, as you can urine, by contracting your muscles. The appearance of the fluid also means that labor is not far off. Contractions will probably start within a few days. Often they start that very day.

The surest sign of labor is steady contractions. You may have recognized what are called Braxton Hicks contractions throughout your pregnancy or toward the end of it. Named after the doctor who "discovered" them, Braxton Hicks contractions are uterine contractions, but they are not the contractions of labor if they don't occur *with increasing intensity* and with enough frequency to bring on birth. If you have recognized Braxton Hicks contractions, then you may know how to recognize early labor contractions, although sometimes real labor is felt in a different place from Braxton Hicks contractions. In that case labor contractions may not be immediately recognizable. To some women they feel like menstrual cramps. To some they feel like constipation, except the sensation periodically deepens. Sometimes the sensation may spread around the thighs and through the abdomen.

It is a myth that in real labors contractions always occur at regular intervals. This is true most of the time, but it is also possible to have real labor with contractions occurring at irregular intervals. You may have a contraction now, the next one five minutes from now, the next one ten minutes after that, the next one three minutes after that, and then one seven minutes later. This may be characteristic of your whole labor. (And Braxton Hicks contractions may occur at regular intervals throughout the day, but fade away by evening.) The tip-off, then, to real labor is *increasing intensity* of contractions. This is also usually accompanied by each contraction lasting longer and longer over time and may be accompanied by decreasing intervals between contractions. If this is what is happening to you and you have been pregnant for about forty weeks, you are probably about to have your baby.

If you are experiencing "back labor" you will probably perceive your contractions as a deepening of constant lower back pressure. Whether you have "back" or "front" labor is a consequence of the position of the baby's head, which is probably due to the shape of your pelvis. If the crown (the hard part towards the back of the top of the head) of the baby's head is rubbing by your lower spine, this is called the posterior position, and you will perceive it as "back labor." Although all vertex (head-down) presentations are normal, anterior presentations are more common than posterior. If you have a posterior presentation, you will probably require a lot more hands-on support from your labor partner, particularly in the way of strong counterpressure, and your labor will probably take longer because the head usually first rotates from a posterior to an anterior presentation.

The length of your labor is individual, no matter what the position of your baby's head. There is a great range in the duration of normal labor, from a precipitous fifteen-minute labor to the three-day labor. All of these can have normal outcomes. As long as the vital signs of both of you are good, the time your labor takes must be normal for this labor. Sometimes, when we read about time boundaries for labor, we are reading a hospital-based doctor's review of how long a labor is allowed to progress, in that hospital, before intervention to speed up labor is introduced.

Complications of Labor

If your first sign of labor has been the breaking of the bag of waters and if labor contractions don't begin within twenty-four hours, almost all doctors and many midwives believe that labor should be induced. This is not to prevent a "dry birth," as some parents believe, because the woman's body continues to produce more fluid for the baby in the uterus. The reason is that statistically there is an increased chance of infection the longer the baby remains in the uterus after the bag has ruptured. To decrease the risk of infection after your waters break, you should not take a bath or have intercourse or introduce any foreign objects such as a tampon through the vagina. Even the birth attendant's gloved fingers increase the risk of infection. However, an internal examination may be medically necessary at some time after the membranes rupture to determine if any dilatation has taken place.

Induced Labor

The decision on whether to go to the hospital to be induced, usually by *Pitocin,* if contractions have not begun within twenty-four hours after the membranes have ruptured, is ultimately yours. Your birth attendant will probably have listened to the fetal heart tones and perhaps be able to offer other factors as evidence for whether you should be induced at the hospital. Doctors usually recommend that you go to the hospital even if labor has begun after the membranes have ruptured and the contractions have slowed down or stopped.

Nonmedical ways to revive or enhance labor include walking around, squatting, nipple stimulation from the partner or breast pump, cuddling, an enema, or removal of a person causing stress.

The doctor projects that waiting for contractions to pick up again will mean a lapse of more than twenty-four hours. Women and birth attendants who take on the responsibility for the increased chance of infection and who stay home anyway, if all other signs are normal, find that the labor picks up again and eventually culminates in birth, even if contractions stop and start again for more than a day. The baby is usually born without infection, since a strong effort is made not to introduce any. At the hospital, frequent examinations, shaving, and the likely introduction of electrodes for internal monitoring, all in a foreign environment, are factors which probably contribute to the increased chance of infection. Before any decision is made to proceed with a home birth after any deviation from the normal, there must be an intelligent determination that all other vital signs of the mother and baby point to a healthy outcome.

Early or Late

If you begin labor earlier than thirty-seven weeks or later than forty-three weeks, you also may not want to have your baby at home. Babies born earlier than full maturity have a statistically lower rate of survival, because usually their life support systems—their respiratory and digestive systems—are not fully developed. They may have a better chance of surviving in the hospital where there is more sophisticated equipment to help them perform these life functions. However, if your premature or early-for-dates baby is born in the hospital and appears to be healthy, you may want to take the baby with you when you are ready to go home, even if the baby hasn't reached the hospital's magic number of 5 lb. Studies have shown that healthy premature babies, even as small as 3 lb., gain weight faster and stay healthy if they are breastfed at home by their mothers. Breast milk is the ideal food for "premies" because of its easy digestibility and immunological properties. Many hospitals allow a mother to bring her milk to the hospital for the baby and allow the parents to touch the baby even if she or he has to stay in an incubator. Some allow the mother to come to the hospital and nurse the baby there. But if your baby is healthy enough for you to do this, you will probably want to take her or him home. In a 1985 study reported in the *New England Journal of Medicine,* an experimental group of premature babies born at the University of Pennsylvania Medical School's hospital were released sooner than the usual protocol and had just as good outcomes as babies subject to the usual longer wait to be released.[1]

If you have followed good prenatal care that emphasized quality nutrition, you will probably not have your baby prematurely. But if you do begin labor a few weeks before your due date, you need not have an overriding concern about the baby being underweight or unhealthy.

On the other hand, if your baby is postmature, there is the danger that the placenta may not continue to function efficiently. At this point, many doctors want women to undergo a nonstress test: the woman goes to the hospital and is attached to the electronic fetal monitor where her contractions are monitored for about a half hour. In a stress test, the woman is also monitored but while she is receiving *Pitocin*. An alternative to this type of testing is an estriol test in which the level of estriol (a hormone produced by the placenta) in the blood is measured every other day or so. Some women consider this more invasive but less risky. In any case, if you are two weeks past your due date, you and your birth attendant will probably want to discuss the possibility of encouraging labor contractions. This doesn't have to be done by artificially rupturing the membranes or administering intravenous *Pitocin* in the hospital. It can be done more gently and with somewhat less risk though a little less surely by achieving orgasm, slightly manipulating the cervix, or other nonmedical practices like taking a bumpy car ride.

These practices may be less risky than artificial rupture or intravenous *Pitocin,* but they probably have some risk also. Of course, these risks must be weighed against the possible risk of not doing anything. If the vital signs are fine, it may still be safest to wait it out. Check back and make sure the due date wasn't miscalculated. The formula for determining the due date is date of start of last menstrual period, minus three months, plus seven days. Maybe the last menstrual period was not a true period, or maybe it wasn't written down or remembered correctly. As long as the vital signs of the baby and mother are good, it is important to remember that fetuses can't read calendars. Your baby doesn't know when you and your doctor decided she or he should be born. Babies come out when they are ready, not necessarily when you are. No one knows for sure what triggers labor. Perhaps what is really annoying you are the daily phone calls from certain people asking if you are "still around."

WHEN TO CALL YOUR BIRTH ATTENDANT

Unless your early signs of labor occur in the middle of the night when most people are asleep, it is considerate to alert your birth attendant to any preliminary activity you recognize. If you are having your baby in the hospital, it doesn't matter as much to your doctor if you call him when contractions are ten minutes apart or even closer together, since most doctors don't plan to go to the hospital until birth is imminent. Even if they get stuck in traffic and miss the birth entirely, the resident can always deliver. But you want a specific person to attend your birth. Especially if you will be using a lay midwife who may not own an electronic beeper or who may be planning to spend the afternoon in the park with her children, it is sensible to call. You may only be saying, "I just want to let you know I had a bloody show. No contractions yet, but maybe you should hold off if you planned an all-day trip today." Also, many home birth attendants realize the importance of being with you for as much of the labor as possible, so they will appreciate an early call.

The birth attendant may come right away, examine you, and leave if you are barely dilated and if it is your first child. But if your contractions slow down or disappear, call your midwife back to your home. Then if labor picks up again after she arrives, you can both surmise that it is your confidence in her presence that helps you to labor along better. Sometimes the birth attendant has to honor a prior commitment or be with family first, but she should try not to leave you once she arrives and you are in labor.

Activities During Labor

Whether the midwife is there or not, continue doing whatever you were doing before you realized you were in labor. This includes housework, local shopping, or walking around. Of course, if your membranes have ruptured you will want to confine yourself to your home so you don't drip over other people's property. At home you may want to make "pathways" with newspapers or old rags and towels if you are leaking amniotic fluid. There are two good reasons for continuing to move around for as long as you can in labor. One is that the activity keeps your mind off the discomfort of your contractions. The other is that the vertical position of your body, with gravity, helps move the baby down toward the vagina.

Your body will tell you when it is time to cease ordinary activity and concentrate on your labor. When you can no longer move about freely and have to stay in one spot, do sit, but remember not to lie down flat on your back, a physiologically bad position for labor. Sit up if you can, so you will feel more alert and can continue to take advantage of gravity. You can bend forward spread-eagled over pillows, kneel with your head resting on the side of a bed, stand and lean on your husband, or lie on your side if you have to lie down. If you can, walk around between contractions.

In sum, a woman may labor in whatever position she is most comfortable. One of the advantages of laboring at home is that you can assume whatever position you like and change as often as you need and not worry about whether the intern thinks it's ladylike to be up on your knees with palms on the floor as if you were about to crawl around. (That happens to be one position to assume to take pressure off your lower back if you are experiencing "back labor.") During labor at home you may do anything else you wish to make yourself comfortable. You may eat, keeping in mind that as labor progresses digestion all but stops, so you won't want heavy foods sitting in your stomach pressing next to the contracting uterus and causing you discomfort. If your membranes have not ruptured, you may want to take a bath or shower in early labor to help relax. At home you can also sing or even dance to your contractions, talk on the phone, or play card games—whatever you like that will make labor pleasant. One thing to be sure to try to do during labor is to urinate every two hours. A full bladder interferes with labor progress. And to help your urine flow and keep you well hydrated, drink fluids often too.

FIRST STAGE LABOR: EFFACEMENT AND DILATATION

As the uterus contracts, it first effaces (thins out) the cervix, or opening of the womb. The cervix also must dilate (widen) enough for the baby's head to pass through. Many times effacement and dilatation have begun as the result of Braxton Hicks contractions, without your being aware. The dilatation of the cervix is measured in centimeters. Your birth attendant will probably examine you to determine how dilated you are. Ten cm. is approximately the width of a newborn baby's head and is called "full dilatation."

In general, you probably won't experience much discomfort for the first few centimeters' dilatation. The contractions leading to 4-6 cm., however, are sometimes known as heavy or active labor. It is around this time that labor will probably start to require your full attention and you will need to concentrate on your relaxation.

TRANSITION

Dilatation from 7 to 10 cm. is called transition, because it marks the passage from labor to birth. It is usually the shortest part of dilatation, but it is also often the most intense because the contractions, if no drugs have been taken, are very efficient. Sometimes transition contractions are run-on and irregular. The baby's head is also passing near the rectum which may cause lower back pain. Many women find that transition is the hardest part of labor and the time they most appreciate having a knowledgeable labor assistant. If transition is discouraging you, your birth attendant and husband should be right there reminding you with eye-to-eye contact that transition is short and that it means your baby will be born soon. Transition may last around an hour. The preceding stage may last at least a few hours and usually longer.

Before you reach full dilatation, you should have located yourself in the place where you want to give birth—at 10 cm. you probably won't feel like moving around. When the cervix is opened to this point, it is wide enough for the baby's head to pass through and into the vagina, or birth canal. More often than not, you will feel like pushing the baby along with each contraction. As long as the cervix is fully dilated, there is no problem with your helping to push the baby through it and on out toward the exit from your body. If you push when the cervix is not fully dilated the baby's head may cause it to become irritated and swollen, making it more difficult for the head to come through, even at full dilatation.

However, if the urge to push is irresistible before 10 cm., it probably won't harm your cervix if you push *gently*. In the hospital, many women are urged to "Push! Push! Push!" as if the staff were a cheering squad. This type of pushing, usually accompanied by breath holding, may irritate the cervix. Really, the uterus could accomplish birth on its own without any strenuous effort on the mother's part, especially if she is in a vertical birth position. No woman should push if she doesn't feel like it, unless there is a medical reason to rush the birth; and even with the urge to push present, gentle pushing, "breathing out the baby," is probably all that is necessary.

EXPULSION

It's a good idea to keep your mouth open while pushing. The effect is to help keep your cervix and vagina loose. Instead of just letting your mouth hang, try singing, smiling, or making noises. Some uninhibited women allow themselves the pleasure of many noises while pushing. It expresses the sexuality of childbirth and gives an outlet to some of the energy they are expending. The expulsion stage usually lasts from about fifteen minutes to two hours. Think "up and out" while pushing and push *gently*. It is not the same kind of pushing as a bowel movement, as some male doctors have told us. Visualizing the baby's head moving down and out the birth canal as the vagina flowers open and mentally or verbally welcoming the baby with each expulsion contraction both help the woman to focus on the correct pushing posture.

You can assume any position that makes you comfortable for birth. The most common position of choice in this country is to sit on a bed, lean back against pillows on a hard wall or backboard, with knees up, feet flat and spread apart on the bed. But you may also prefer to lie on your side, squat, or get up on hands and knees. It is even possible to stand and lean or stand and squat to give birth. Both a full squat and a standing squat widen the pelvis up to 2 cm. If you choose a certain position where your birth attendant can't see the baby coming out, she may ask you to change to an alternative position. A position where she can see better may also make it easier to administer a perineal massage, which some midwives do to keep the area stimulated with blood, reducing the chance of tearing. However, if the position the midwife suggests is not comfortable, she should be accommodating.

It is hard to offer estimates on the average length of the expulsion stage of labor, because so much of what is considered average is what is usual for a hospital delivery, where expediency is often the rule. The expulsion stage may be several minutes or it may last as long as an hour or two. Of course, if it lasts many hours and no progress is being made, hospitalization is necessary because there is probably a physiological reason for the delay. But as long as the vital signs are normal, there is no need to speed the birth. A woman in this situation would want to do a lot of walking around so gravity and motion can help the baby's head come down.

It is actually advantageous to have the head born slowly, because that, too, decreases the possibility of tearing. It also decreases the possibility of shocking the new being into earth and makes for a smoother adjustment to the change of environment. If you feel the urge to push once you are fully dilated, remember to push gently and gradually. Pushing will be most effective if you wait until each contraction starts to peak and you can feel the baby moving in the birth canal with each push. On the other hand, some women would rather push between contractions and blow during them.

BIRTH

When the baby's head is about to emerge into the world, you will probably feel a tight, burning sensation around your vagina. It might feel as if it is bursting apart and, indeed, it is stretching more than it ever has before. But your body has prepared itself for such stretching. And if the skin around the vagina looks taut and pale, your birth attendant may massage the blood back into the area. If you do tear, anyway, it will probably not hurt, since the baby's head is also pressing on the nerve endings there. The tear, if it occurs, will probably be much slighter than what you are imagining by the burning, stretching feeling you are experiencing. Sheila Kitzinger, in her 1981 study on episiotomy, found tearing preferable to cutting in terms of postpartum complications to the mother.[2]

As the head is actually being born, it is best not to push, to minimize the effects on both you and your baby. The birth attendant will support the head at this time to ease the baby's exit. Although the emphasis is on slowness and gentleness, this may be an ecstatic moment for you. It was meant to be. If it is your first child, at no time since your own birth have you been so close to this rite of passage. You share it with every mother who has ever lived and every mother who ever shall live. It is an act so often repeated, so common, but with sensations so vibrant that newness and uniqueness are discovered each time. You may wish to reach down and touch the baby's sticky wet head as it is emerging. You may be lucky enough to hear the baby's first breath, ending in a noisy exhalation known as the first cry, before the body is even out. Some babies wait until they are completely out and then start breathing.

The rest of the body will probably come out on the contraction after the head is born. The shoulders are born one at a time, not simultaneously. If a shoulder does not come out on the contraction after the head is born, the birth attendant might ask for special assistance from you in the way of proper pushing. Once the shoulders are born, the rest of the baby's body usually comes out with very little effort on your part because it is thinner than the head and slippery.

CARE FOR YOUR NEWBORN

Since your baby has had no depressing medication from your bloodstream, he will probably start breathing immediately. If not, the birth attendant will take steps to encourage the baby. As long as the umbilical cord is still attached and working and the baby starts to *move*, there is no need for you to panic if your baby does not begin breathing immediately, even if it takes a few minutes.

Breastfeeding

After your baby is all out and breathing on her own, the birth attendant will put the baby in your arms or lay her across your belly. If left on your body, the new baby may actually squirm up on its own and find your nipple. If you are holding your baby, she will enjoy looking at your face and feeling your touch as you stroke her cheek and hearing your gentle words as you speak. (You will discover that newborn infants do, indeed, see and hear.) Unless the room is very warm, your birth attendant will probably place a cover over you both. Since new babies are both naked and wet, they could get chilled. Covering the baby's head will help to maintain body temperature. If you move your baby to your breast, she will probably begin to suck, although some babies prefer to just smell and lick for a while. The baby should be encouraged to breastfeed by the end of the first hour after birth, to establish the sucking response and to help your uterus contract.

Cutting The Cord

The umbilical cord need not be cut—ever (it would rot and fall off within a week), except that it is awkward to keep it attached. Delaying cord clamping and cutting, at least until the cord stops pulsating, allows the baby a smooth transition in sources of sustenance. Cutting it too soon also denies the baby its full share of blood. It must be cut immediately only if it is extremely short, which is rare, or if there is a certain type of blood incompatibility. It is also not necessary to clean off the baby thoroughly. If the baby has difficulty breathing, the birth attendant will suction out some mucus from his respiratory tract. If the baby is covered with mucus and blood, the birth attendant will likewise do some wiping. But the white substance covering the baby's body, called vernix, should be left on because it protects the baby's skin. If you like, you can rub it into the baby's skin or you can let it get absorbed by itself.

Birth of the Placenta

As the birth attendant looks over the baby, she will also be keeping an eye on you. She will be watching for the appearance of your placenta and checking to see if you have excessive bleeding or lacerations. Tearing requiring stitches is not common, but some midwives don't stitch, so you may have to contact a doctor in that situation. Hemorrhage, also not common, is usually treated successfully at home if it is not severe. The placenta will probably appear within twenty minutes of the baby's birth and is only cause for concern if it does not come out after more than an hour or if it is not whole when it does come out.

UNATTENDED HOME BIRTH

Many husbands, including those whose wives plan hospital births, wonder what they should do if birth comes quicker than the birth attendant. If you are planning a home birth, this is an even more distinct possibility, though still an uncommon one if the birth attendant is given enough notice. It is important for your mate to remember that there is very little more to be done other than being the loving labor coach. Probably the best physical help to you and the baby would be massage, especially if the skin around the vagina appears taut and pale, and support of the baby's head by a firm hold as it emerges from the vagina. If your husband is too nervous to assume any part of the birth attendant's job, let him continue to give you emotional support and encourage you to relax and let your body do its job. Make sure you are well placed on a big area, so the baby will have plenty of space to slide out and rest between your legs. If the birth attendant still hasn't arrived by the time the cord has stopped pulsating, your partner may boil two shoelaces and tie them one inch apart, a few inches from the baby. Snip the cord in between the two laces with a boiled scissors. Or if he's still nervous, the cord can just remain there for hours till you or some-one else cuts it.

HANDLING YOUR NEW BABY

Some couples wonder whether they should make a special effort to incorporate the ideas of Frederick Leboyer into their home birth. Leboyer is the French physician who believes in minimizing the trauma of birth for the baby with soft lights, silence, a massage, and a bath. The publicity given the Leboyer method is well deserved if it causes the medical profession and parents to ask, "How does it seem to the baby to be born?" "How can we alter the hospital environment to make birth less traumatic for the baby?" But, as Dr. Leboyer would seem to have it, judging from his book and film, the doctor massages the baby after birth, the doctor bathes the baby who, in the film, is moving his lips as if he would rather nurse, and the doctor teaches the mother the proper way to touch the baby, something she is assumed not to know.[3] There is some controversy in hospital delivery rooms about dimming lights and wheeling in bathtubs. Some modern doctors "allow" their patients to deliver à la Leboyer. It seems that, first, doctors took our babies away; now some say we can have them back. Somehow, before hospitalization, mothers knew what to do with a newborn baby without special instruction from a male doctor. Of course, in your own home, you can give your baby as many relaxing baths as you wish. But do you think this is what you'll feel like doing after she or he is born? You can be sure that the atmosphere of a home birth will do much to minimize the trauma of birth for the baby without any special effort.

The best things to do after the baby is born are whatever seems natural to do. After you and the baby have been checked over and wiped, you will probably just want to continue getting acquainted with each other sensually. Try for some time alone for the new baby and both parents and possibly the siblings, without the midwife and others. Within an hour after birth you may feel like showering, changing clothes, and eating. Or you may not. You should surely be offered food and, if you are not hungry, at least take some juice for energy and replacement of fluids.

TAKE CARE OF YOURSELF AFTER BIRTH

Do try to urinate as soon as possible after birth. If you are still unable to urinate after twelve hours, call your birth attendant. Also, if your baby hasn't urinated after twelve hours, call the midwife or doctor. But with frequent breastfeeding the baby will probably urinate before that time. It is important to nurse the baby often. The colostrum, or yellowish premilk, is rich in antibodies for the baby and helps to flush out any mucus. The frequent sucking stimulates your uterus to contract, sometimes vigorously, which contributes to the prevention of hemorrhage. The birth attendant will probably stay around for a few hours after birth to make sure your uterus is contracting satisfactorily. And if she is not qualified to do thorough newborn examinations, she may suggest a home visit from a phsyician. In the interim, you should know that the baby's first bowel movement (meconium) will be sticky and blackish. And your baby may not sleep as much as you expected but may yawn or sneeze a lot and breathe somewhat irregularly.

Guests at a birth are just as happy to party without the new parents present. If you would rather rest with the new baby, inform your birth attendant and she can see that the celebration moves away from your room. If everyone wants to hold the baby, you need not allow it. The baby may actually be upset by so much handling. After you, the next person to hold the baby should be the father, and then the siblings or other people as close as siblings, providing you want to let them and your baby doesn't seem to mind.

Beyond these, there are very few, if any, "shoulds." The demands of labor behind you, the beauty of a home birth is that it is now your experience to keep. After the birth is a time for the new baby and the family to rest, relax, get acquainted, talk about the birth, and establish foundations—together. Take the phone off the hook or refuse guests if you wish. You need answer only to one another. The demands of modern existence will force you to deal with the outside world soon enough. So adore each other wholly while you can.

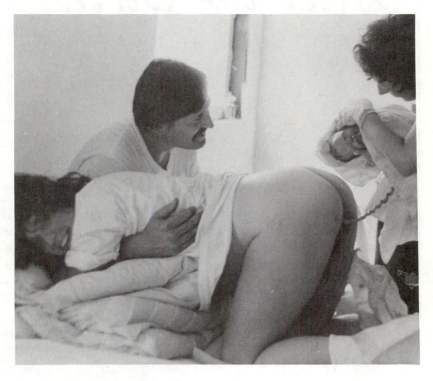

Byron Greatorex photograph

CHAPTER 8

"After the Birth"

How you care for your new baby, including your style of infant feeding and mothering, are choices only you can make. For too long in our society mothers have been regarded as mostly incapable of making important decisions regarding their children. The implications are twofold: that anyone else (kind aunt, baby nurse) could do the job just as well, if not better, and that an authority must be consulted for the answer to any question that arises. Lesser authorities answer most of our questions by advising, "Ask your doctor." Then, when we go to this highest authority, the doctor jokes about the crazy lady who keeps calling to ask about the color of her baby's bowel movement.

In truth, there is no one who could tell you the right thing to do concerning your child, a unique individual whom *you* know better than anyone else. Unless there is a medical problem, the doctor is probably telling you what he would do or did do with his child. The doctor is using the same common sense you could use. Authorities like doctors or books or experienced mothers are

106

sources of information for you, to be drawn on by you as often as you like. But the most important added factor to this information is your own sense of what is best, based on your intimate knowledge of the particular little person who began life as a part of you—and who is still a part of you.

TOGETHER AND APART: BONDING

A young mother with her newborn pressed against her chest in a cloth baby carrier entered a roomful of acquaintances, who commented on how cute the baby was, how nicely he was sleeping, and how much weight the mother had lost. But one newly married man said, "She really looks the same to me. She just moved her bump up."

Infant care may mean "just moving the bump up," or soothing the adjustment to living by meeting the baby's needs outside the womb in a way that simulates life inside it, but most medical professionals in this country seem to be unaware of this. It is surprising that so little research has been done in the area of human mother-child bonding and effects of its lack: separating the mother and her newborn ranks first among unnatural practices in routine medical care. Probably one reason for the paucity of research is that behaviorism as a science had not developed one hundred years ago and earlier when most births occurred at home. When the importance of psychological experimentation became more widely accepted, it already seemed normal to have babies in hospitals. Still, it is strange that students of psychology study what happens when we separate offspring from geese or rats or monkeys or kangaroos—but it is only recently that we have observed that human mothers and babies also seem to exhibit species-specific mother-child bonding behavior. Marshall Klaus of Case Western Reserve University has identified some of these behaviors: picking up the baby and establishing eye contact, talking to the baby in a high-pitched voice, stroking the baby's cheek with the fingertips, touching the baby's extremities with the fingertips and then the baby's trunk with a massaging, encompassing motion of the palms, and putting the baby to the breast where the baby may lie for a while before sucking.[1] According to observation by other researchers as well, there is also a "dance" between mother and newborn, a coordinated motor interaction between the two which includes the brand-new baby actually moving in rhythm with the mother's speaking pattern. There is also some indication that the atmosphere of euphoria or excitement surrounding a home birth, which is often absent in a hospital birth, may have significant implications for all involved. It appears certain from the research of Klaus that complex interactions between mother and child are necessary for the survival of the infant.

This work confirms the intuition of many home birth couples: that the baby should not be separated from the mother in the crucial hours after birth. The most cruel punishment of all, separating a new life from its only source of love for hours on end, has been practiced in our society for years, without considering its possible effects. Now that we live in a society where rape and other violent crimes are on the increase, where divorce and the dissolution of families are common, and where "communications gaps" between parents and teenagers are almost expected, some behaviorists are beginning to wonder whether everything might have been handled wrong from the start—the start being birth.

One social scientist who recognized early in his career the importance of satisfying the tactile needs of the human child is anthropologist Ashley Montagu. He has shown how maternal deprivation may actually result in the physical, mental, and emotional retardation of the offspring. Montagu states that the main difference between humans and other mammals is the size and development of the human brain. On a scale with other mammals, the human gestation period should be longer than it is, but it is only nine months, because if the fetus's head were to continue at its rate of development, it would be too big to be born. Therefore, Montagu says, the human baby is born, but gestation continues outside the uterus for about another six months. It is only at that time that the baby ceases to be totally dependent on the mother and is able to move around away from her. Montagu thinks that the continuing needs of the fetus can be met exterogestatively through touch, that the importance of touch on human development has been ignored for too long, and that denying babies skin contact after birth may affect them in ways that are not often correctable.[2]

Until these factors are more completely understood and, more significantly, until the effects of inhibiting the development of these bonding mechanisms are understood, you who are having your baby at home can be happy that you are providing yourself and your baby with the normal atmosphere for optimum development. Klaus' work not only provides increasing evidence on the value of home birth (although he personally doesn't endorse it) but also helps hospitals change their policies on allowing parents to care for normal full-term infants and also premature or otherwise hospitalized newborns. Aberrations of maternal behavior, including the battered child syndrome, are known to be higher among mothers of premature and sick infants who have undergone prolonged hospitalization and who have been denied early tactile contact.

Contact

So just moving the bump up *is* what infant care is about. Newborn babies love to snuggle close, nurse frequently, be carried about, and touch skin-to-skin. It seems many times as if they wish they could return to the comfort and security of the uterus. But since they can't, it is the job of the mother, as much as she can, to simulate life in utero by meeting the needs of the baby as wholly as possible outside it. Then one day, when the security and love she has provided have guided the baby through the gradual adjustment to extrauterine life, the baby's head will pull away from her breast, the arms from her chest, and the baby will crawl away, walk away, the child will run away, and the adult will move away. Each step in its own time.

Breastfeeding is so much a part of quality mothering that most home birth services include intention to nurse the baby as a prerequisite for their assistance at the birth. Since one reason most couples choose home birth is to give the baby the best possible start in life, it is rare to find a home birth mother who doesn't extend this desire to breastfeeding. Although it is possible to rear babies satisfactorily by bottlefeeding, there are many reasons why breastfeeding is better for you and your baby.

Breastfeeding

One of the main advantages of breastfeeding for the mother is that the sucking action causes the uterus to contract. Early and frequent breastfeeding after birth reduces both the chance of hemorrhage for the mother and the amount of blood lost. Another effect of the contracting action caused by breastfeeding is that it is easier for you to return to your pre-pregnancy figure. Additionally, some studies report a positive correlation between the length of time spent breastfeeding and decreased incidence of breast cancer. Breastfeeding may also act as a natural child spacer if you are not interested in using mechanical birth control right after the birth or at all. This means that if you breastfeed without supplementation (no water, no formula, no solid food) for at least the first six months of the baby's life, your menstrual periods probably won't resume for from six to fifteen months after birth. Since a woman's first period following birth almost always has *not* been preceded by ovulation, a new mother is usually, *but not always,* incapable of becoming pregnant until menstruation resumes. Finally, many mothers like the feeling of confidence breastfeeding gives them. There is satisfaction in knowing that you yourself are still capable of totally nourishing your baby and meeting her needs.

The advantages to the baby are many. Most important, mother's milk is the food most ideally suited to the baby. It is human milk for a human baby. A mother cat would not think of feeding her kitten dog's milk: why let a cow provide the food for your baby? Human milk for human babies means that everything in your milk is in exactly the right proportion for your baby and perfectly suited. Cans of formula wouldn't state that they are "closest to" or "nearest to" mother's milk if they could say "exactly like." One reason they can't is that certain properties of human milk are still being discovered. When bottlefeeding was very popular some babies died on a formula diet; the formula lacked vitamin E. Now vitamin E is in formula, but who knows what else is missing?

Because you are feeding your baby the ideally suited food, he will not be allergic to your milk. Diaper rash and the kind of persistent crankiness known as colic are possible allergic reactions to cow's milk formulas. Sometimes babies are so allergic to cow's milk formulas that they become severely dehydrated and have to be hospitalized while many different types of formulas are tried. Cow's milk curds may be too large for the baby's digestive system. These problems don't occur with breast milk.

Occasionally a very sensitive baby will show a reaction to a particular food the mother has eaten usually in large quantity. In this case, the mother can eliminate that food from her diet for a while and try it again when the baby gets older and a little more tolerant. An example of such a food would be cow's milk in a mother's diet. You don't need to drink milk to make milk anyway, and there are other good sources of protein, calcium, and fluids.

Mother's milk is always at the right temperature and easily available; you can't run out of it if the drugstore closes or you're stuck in traffic. It doesn't smell or stain badly like formula when it is spit up or eliminated in a bowel movement. Also, there is growing evidence that formula feeding could lead to lifelong obesity, while breastfed babies usually become lean and muscular toddlers and children and will remain that way as long as their diets stay healthy.

Along with fewer digestive upsets, there are fewer skin disorders and diaper rashes and fewer respiratory upsets and other sicknesses. Recent studies have shown colostrum and breast milk to have a low pH factor, preventing growth of pathogenic E. coli. There is also evidence that breastfeeding helps prevent later orthodontal problems because of the kind of jaw development fostered by this particular kind of sucking.

In addition to making you feel good about continuing to provide for your baby, breastfeeding and the kind of closeness that results also make the baby feel secure and loved. Breastfeeding also saves time, since there is no preparation of formula, and it saves money. You don't have to introduce other foods for at least the first half of the first year of life, which also decreases the chance of allergies and digestive upsets.

Begin nursing your baby within the first hour after birth, if not immediately after. Hold the baby in the traditional rock-a-bye-baby position with your nipple touching the baby's cheek. A baby is born with a rooting reflex and will turn his face to your breast once it is felt on the cheek. Don't squeeze the baby's cheeks, or let anyone else do this, in an attempt to turn his face toward you; the baby may become confused, since both cheeks are being touched. You may have to cup your breast with thumb on top and other fingers below to direct the nipple between the baby's lips. Although your baby's mouth is small and your breast may be large, try to get as much of the areola (darker area) into the baby's mouth as possible. This helps prevent soreness from the baby chewing on just the tip of the nipple and also allows sucking on the main milk ducts around the areola. Hold the baby securely so her or his head doesn't keep slipping back. Recent research, as reported in the *Journal of the Nurses Association of the American College of Obstetricians and Gynecologists* (1985) shows that the best way to prevent nipple soreness is to hold the baby really horizontally, belly to belly, as if both of the baby's knees touched the nonnursing nipple. Sometimes a pillow or two on your lap helps raise the baby to the right level. The baby's ear should be toward the ceiling.

It is important for the baby to get the colostrum that is in the breast right after birth. In addition to providing immunities, it is rich in protein. Colostrum also has a laxative effect, helping to clean the meconium out of the baby's body and preparing the digestive tract for the true white milk. If this is not your first baby, these early nursings may cause you to feel strong cramps in your belly. Your uterus must contract after birth, and the sucking action on your breast helps it along. If the contractions feel painful, take deep, slow, relaxing breaths. The contractions probably won't be felt more than a couple of days. If this is your first baby, you probably won't feel the contractions.

Nurse the baby as frequently as you can, at least every two hours unless the baby is sleeping. Don't let the baby go for more than four hours without a feeding in the daytime. Frequent nursing helps prevent the breasts from becoming engorged when the true milk comes in. After a home birth and the frequent nursing which accompanies it, milk may begin to appear twenty-four hours after birth. If you do get engorged, you may have to hand express a little milk so the nipple protrudes enough for your baby to latch on. If you are uncomfortably full, remember this condition usually lasts only about a day, and your baby is the best pump.

After your milk comes in, continue to nurse frequently. Most new babies want to nurse approximately every two hours. This means that while the baby may sleep for four or five hours sometimes (at night, you hope), she may want to nurse more often than every two hours at other times. It is better to look upon each nursing session as part of a growing relationship and not just a feeding. Then the clock won't be so important; the baby can't read it anyway. Just nurse your baby whenever it seems appropriate. You don't have to worry about overfeeding unless you have been nursing practically nonstop for hours, which sometimes happens, and the baby is vomiting. Try to give both breasts equal stimulation at each nursing session. Aim for at least ten minutes on each side, and try to alternate which side you begin on.

Frequent nursing also helps guarantee that the baby is getting enough, which is a concern of many people. Be confident that breastfeeding works on a supply-and-demand basis, and the more you nurse the more milk you will have. The best way to know that the baby is getting enough is to let him nurse on demand—which usually averages out to every two hours—and count wet diapers, if you are in doubt. It your baby has at least six wet diapers a day (the bowel movement schedule varies greatly with breastfed babies, so we are just talking about urine here), there is probably adequate milk production. Sometimes it is hard to tell wetness with some kinds of disposable diapers, so you may want to switch to cloth for a few days if you are anxious to test this out. If your baby is not nursing as often as every two hours but still has lots of wet diapers, you can also be confident.

If you are giving the baby water, this rule doesn't hold since some of the urine is not from your milk. A breastfed infant doesn't need water or any other supplements. There is enough water in the milk. Giving water just weighs on the baby's stomach and may fill up the baby so much that she doesn't want to breastfeed. There is also the bother of preparing unnecessary bottles, which may introduce air bubbles (gas) and give the baby nipple confusion. You are the one who will probably be more thirsty, since your body is being emptied of fluids. You will probably want to drink more than usual. Juices are healthiest, but you can just drink extra water if you are concerned about your weight.

You also don't have to wash your breasts before or after feedings. Too much water has a dishpan-hand effect on your nipples. Stop using soap entirely, as it tends to be drying. A shower once a day is enough wetness for your nipples. They secrete their own hormone which cleans them. Leaving them exposed to the air as much as possible also toughens them and helps prevent soreness. You can use pure hydrous lanolin on sore nipples, which you won't have to wipe off before the baby nurses.

If you want to break the suction when the baby is nursing, gently slip your finger in the corner of the baby's mouth. Some breastfed babies have to be burped, and others don't. Don't take birth control pills when you're breastfeeding, and check with your doctor and La Leche League about any other medications that are prescribed for you. Know that the baby's bowel movement will be approximately the color and consistency of mustard. It is normal for a breastfed baby to have a bowel movement seven times a day or every seven days. Constipation and diarrhea are indicated by the consistency, not the frequency, of movements, and there will be no painfully hard little balls if the baby is on mother's milk only.

There is usually no need to introduce supplements of any kind for the first six months of life. Most babies are just not ready for supplements sooner, and early introduction may actually cause problems. You, the mother, however, may take vitamins or other supplements, if your diet isn't adequate.

If you don't want to leak milk in front of other people, you can discreetly press on your nipples when you feel the milk start to come out. Leaking has to do with sphincter muscle control and not milk supply, so don't panic if you don't leak ever, or if you used to leak or feel engorged and now your body has adjusted. The baby will go through growth spurts at around five or six weeks, at around three months, and at about six months. During these times, the baby will nurse more frequently for a few days, building up your milk supply to meet the increased demand. For night feedings, take the baby in to bed with you so you can continue to get some rest.

If you have any questions or problems about breastfeeding, from advice on nursing discreetly to what to do about a clogged milk duct, phone a La Leche League volunteer. They are the breast-feeding experts. It is good to start attending their monthly meetings while you are pregnant, but you can also start going after the baby is born. Free literature, a lending library, and discussions providing information and support are available.

As La Leche League says, breastfeeding is not complicated; society's attitude toward it makes it complicated. The worst but most frequent advice you will receive will come from people who have never breastfed successfully or who think "suck" is a dirty word. You know what is best for your baby in terms of the nursing relationship and the period of adjustment you are both undergoing. As long as the baby is gaining weight and is healthy in every other way, you should be satisfied that the breastfeeding is going well. Nurse and hold your baby frequently. A baby left to cry it out only learns that you don't care if she needs someone. You can spoil an older child by catering to whims for material things, but you can never spoil a baby by giving the security of love.

LAWS ABOUT NEWBORNS

As for other areas of newborn care, check with your birth attendant. Ask her if there are any blood tests required by law in your state. It is likely a PKU test is required. It could uncover a factor missing from your baby's blood which could lead to mental retardation if left untreated. Since the treatment involves cessation of breastfeeding and since there are a number of false positives in PKU testing, get at least one retest if your baby comes up positive. If you bring your baby to a government facility for necessary blood tests and inoculations, be aware that some employees here, too, may be anxious to implicate an illegal midwife or otherwise complicate the situation once they learn your baby has been born at home. Remember that you yourself have done nothing illegal by giving birth at home. However, it is required that all births be registered. Your birth attendant will either take care of this for you or, if she wishes to remain anonymous, will discuss with you the course to follow. It also is surely required in your state that your birth attendant put silver nitrate or a substitute in your baby's eyes as a prophylactic treatment for gonorrhea. Silver nitrate initially seems to burn the baby's eyes and affect vision, so it is not a good idea to have it administered in the first hours after birth when you want your baby to see you well. If you are complying with this law, silver nitrate can be administered before the birth attendant goes home. If you and your husband have Rh incompatibility, you will probably want the midwife to put some of the umbilical cord blood in the refrigerator for subsequent testing to determine the baby's blood type. If the mother is Rh negative and the father Rh positive and the baby proves Rh positive, an injection of Rhogam for the mother will prevent a future miscarriage or neonatal death from Rh disease.

Having a pediatrician makes it easier to secure the proper forms for required tests and to administer checkups. But if a private pediatrician is expensive for you, these requirements may also be met at a public health facility.

Circumcision. If you have a boy baby, you will have to decide what to do about a circumcision, since you won't have the option of hospital circumcision. If you are doing it for ritual reasons, that is one matter. But if not, it is important to know that even the American Academy of Pediatrics agrees that there are no health benefits to routine circumcision. Since a boy can learn to care for him uncircumcised penis as easily as learning to brush his teeth, as he gets older, the earlier push toward routine circumcision needs to be reassessed. If you do decide to have your boy circumcised, it is better to have circumcision professional, such as a *mohel,* do the job. A doctor may want to hospitalize your baby, with all that this entails, including anesthesia and risk of infection, unnecessary separation and procedures, and extra expense and trauma. Even if you find a doctor willing to perform a circumcision in his office, his medical background will cause him to perform it as a surgically exact, slow, painful, and traumatic procedure. A *mohel* is quicker, more efficient and experienced, will do the procedure in your home, and will give the baby to you right afterward to nurse. It is wise to follow the Jewish tradition of waiting until the eighth day for the circumcision. Then the baby's supply of vitamin K for clotting reaches a high level, and necessary bonding has already occurred between you and your son. If you do have a circumcision performed, follow the *mohel*'s instructions for keeping the area clean.

Navel. As for the umbilical cord stump, no special procedures need be followed in caring for it. The cord will dry up and fall off by itself. This often occurs in less than a week after home births. If you notice the navel is oozing pus or blood or there is redness encircling it, call your birth attendant or the baby's doctor. Keeping the diaper lower than the navel will help prevent such infection from starting.

Baths. When the navel and penis are clear, it is all right to immerse the baby's body in water. Prior to this, a baby may be wiped with a soft damp cloth or cotton in the creases or other places where she or he is dirty. Oils, lotions, and powders are usually not necessary, except in the treatment of rash. A substance in a powder, such as zinc, may be harmful to the baby if inhaled. When the time comes, your baby may like the free floating feeling of being immersed in water. Some mothers find it is relaxing for both themselves and the baby to take a bath together in the adult tub after a particularly trying day. But it is not necessary to bathe your baby daily or even often if you or the baby don't feel like it. If the baby is perspiring to a point where her hair begins to smell, a bath is usually indicated, but otherwise, since newborns don't play in the mud, they don't need frequent baths to get clean.

Safety. A matter which deserves serious attention is car safety. Holding a baby securely in your arms in a car is not safe. The force of a sudden stop or even minor crash would propel the baby out of your arms at the speed at which your vehicle was going, possibly through the windshield. Merely laying the baby in a car bed is also not safe. A baby should be secured in a government-approved car seat. This is the law in almost every part of the country. If the baby is crying and wants to nurse, pull over to the side of the road and nurse the baby there.

Priorities

Infant care is meeting responsibilities like these, but it is also a state of mind. The hardest part with the first child is the adjustment: one day you are your own person and the next day a whole new other being is totally dependent on you. Even if this is not your first child, your household and life have become accustomed to certain routines which now must be changed. In general, the older must defer to the younger. The adults are supposedly mature persons, capable of understanding reasons for things like why they can't always eat on time. But a new baby is totally incapable of understanding any reason for that. Strangely, some people attribute adult cunning and logic to tiny infants, suggesting the baby purposely wants to be fed just when he knows you are eating, or relaxing, or whatever you are enjoying doing. If you think about these things from the baby's point of view—"I know how I feel now, but how does this seem to the baby?"—your course of action and the direction of your sympathies may be different. A crying baby is a person who is calling out to you because he has an unfulfilled need.

Perhaps the classic study by Rene Spitz will help you to set your priorities. Ninety-one babies from a foundling home were given all the attention thought necessary for survival—diaper changes, correct diet, sterile conditions—but they were denied the affection of their mothers or any one constant person. Thirty-four of the babies died, and most of the others grew up retarded. A control group of babies was cared for by their unmarried and little-educated mothers. No babies died, and development was normal.[3]

Your basic principle should be that people are more important than things. Having a clean house is never more important than sitting down and relaxing with your feet up and your baby on your lap, loved and appreciated for being the unique individual she or he is. Sometimes—especially when you have been awake for fifteen hours or more—it is very hard to have perspective, to see your way clear to things ever being any other way. It is helpful to remember at these moments that time does pass quickly and that it will be a very short time before your baby will be crawling, then walking, then running away from you. Giving your baby a lot of love, attention, and security now is the best way of assuring that one day he will be strong enough to take these steps. We are all human; even the best mothers take a hot "fifteenth-hour shower" while the baby cries. But if your goals are well thought out, you will be able to give good care to your baby most of the time.

Help. If you are unable to put people first at all costs, you might consider getting househould help for a while. You won't need a baby nurse, because all you really need to know is how to stay in bed with the baby and breastfeed and take it easy. La Leche League can answer questions about breastfeeding; a mother at one of their meetings can show you how to fold a diaper, and your common sense can tell you not to make the water too hot if you give the baby a bath. But while you care for your baby in the early weeks it will be relaxing to have someone else do the shopping and essential housework like cooking and washing dishes and clothes. Your mate should be willing to undertake these responsibilities, but if this is not possible, you may have to depend on close friends or, if you feel you must, hire a housekeeper to do this work for you. In some parts of the country, *doula* services have sprung up. *Doula* means, loosely, "mothering the mother." The *doula* comes in and meets the mother's needs through housework and instruction on baby care, but she is also usually an expert on breastfeeding and "talking through" the childbirth experience, which most housekeepers are not, and willing to rub the mother's back or bring the husband's suit to the cleaners, which most baby nurses are not. The modern *doula* replaces the kind aunt or other female relative who filled this role in earlier days, before nuclear families, thousand-mile separations, and employment outside the home for women over 50.

Sometimes close friends or relatives will ask, "Can I help?" meaning, "Can I give the baby a bottle?" You will have to explain that this is not quite the kind of help you were hoping for. Of course, on days when you forget what it was like to have your arms to yourself, it is helpful to have someone else take the baby for a walk around the neighborhood for a half hour or so. It may be a good idea for you to make yourself a mental list of general priorities for the first six months of the baby's life, which may be something like: baby, mother, father, shopping, laundry, cleanup essential for health (wash dishes and toilet), cleanup essential for not insulting company (sweep or vacuum floors once a week).

You see that one of your top priorities is taking care of yourself because you are taking care of the baby. Keeping up a healthy diet goes a long way in keeping yourself feeling good. You don't have to "eat for two" just because you are breastfeeding, if this is your excuse to have two desserts; but you can eat enough to stay healthy and not worry about your weight, since the fully nursing baby will take up to 1,000 calories a day from you. Some new mothers find that meeting the baby's needs and the minimal requirements for cleanliness like clearing the table, showering, and getting dressed can take the whole day to accomplish, and they may actually forget to eat. If you see you don't have time to sit down for a meal, you can keep pieces of cut-up cheese or meat and fruits and vegetables in your refrigerator for snacking throughout the day. If you are eating meals like this, drink juices or milk during the day, not just water. Nutritionist Adelle Davis developed a drink called "pep-up" which you may want to keep handy for sipping.[4] Your added thirst requirements may also be met by drinking herbal teas. Some, like shepherd's purse, have healing properties for after birth.

Your birth attendant can help suggest ways to care for your body. A shower once a day and changing of sanitary pads are usually enough. If you have strong pains, gushes of fresh red blood, or if your discharge smells foul, the birth attendant should be called. It is normal for your discharge to get more mixed with mucus and browner in color as time goes on. This discharge, or lochia, can last anywhere from ten days to six weeks. A good birth attendant will check you over at one-day, one-week, and six-week intervals after the birth—or all three times—to mark your progress. It is a good idea to exercise the perineum. Contract and release the orifices several times each, many times a day, to retone the muscles stretched to capacity during birth. Exercise like sit-ups may be begun slowly, days or a week after birth, depending on your general physical condition. Just raising your head off the bed while lying flat on your back is a good way to start retoning muscles stretched by pregnancy, and if you do progress through "curl-ups" to true sit-ups, remember to bend your knees to prevent lower back injury. Consciousness of the proper way to lift a heavy baby or older child also contributes to preventing back injury. Walking briskly with the baby carriage is also good exercise.

Getting enough rest is an important requirement for after birth. The hard work of giving birth may tire you, as may meeting the needs of a new baby. You can find ways to rest and relax thoughout the day and night even if you don't sleep as many hours total as you did before the baby was born. Nap when the baby naps. This is not usually possible if you have older children. In that case, you can make sure the times you breastfeed the baby are times when you sit down with your feet up and read or talk with your older child. Women who get run-down, which often shows itself in the development of a breast infection, usually are doing too much housework or having too much company or are trying to meet too many responsibilities outside the home too soon.

Outside Work. It is certainly possible to have a new baby, breast-feed, and work outside the home, as more and more women are demonstrating every day. Quality mothering is practiced while the mother and baby are together. While they are not, as close a substitute as possible is found. It is not easy to take on several major commitments at once and do them each well, so ideally priorities have been set before the decision to have a baby was made. There are enough possibilities open to women so that the decision to have a baby should be theirs, with arrangements made to lessen or temporarily postpone for at least a year the commitments to outside work.

Good diet and exercise will help keep you emotionally healthy, too. But there are other considerations over which you have less control. Our society does not always show the required support for new mothers. Babies are not always welcome at restaurants or in an office. Relatives and friends may not be helpful or they may live too far away even to try. And many times your image of being a mother was very different from the way you are feeling now. If you find that you are staying at home for many hours most days and don't like it, your midwife or childbirth education instructor may be helpful in bringing you together with other new mothers of a like philosophy so you can have adult company and conversation while you care for your babies. La Leche League meetings are also good for this.

Personal Life. Your relationship with your mate is important, because he is the person with whom you can share many of your feelings. The kind of husband who is more interested in finding a hot dinner on the table when he comes home than in helping his wife to care for the new baby is becoming a disappearing breed. If you are still married to one of these remnants, however, you will have to discuss priorities with him. If your husband wants to participate as fully as possible in child care, he will need your support as much as you need his, since child care as a legitimate activity for men is still not universally accepted. So communication is important no matter what kind of partner you have.

Sexual relations may be resumed as soon after childbirth as you and your mate desire. A woman usually does not feel like having intercourse until after her perineum no longer feels sore. Communication is also essential here, especially if there is uneasiness about a leaking vagina and breasts. Many couples have discovered the joys of sensual stimulation not culminating in intercourse. Kissing, hugging, and kind words go a long way at a time of your lives punctutated by interrupted sleep and the realization that you no longer have dreamy endless moments to spend with only each other.

Some new fathers are concerned that breastfeeding deprives them of essential child care. If your mate feels this way, think of the many things he can do for his child: changing diapers, giving baths, singing, rocking, and playing are part of child care. Fathers who try can learn ways of relating to their babies that their wives cannot dupliate. A father who relieves his wife of a crying baby who refuses to nurse and takes the baby on a walking tour of the home, softly explaining all the sites until the baby falls asleep on his shoulder, is giving a gift of love to both his wife and his baby. A sensitive father may want to take off his shirt and the baby's and quietly sing the baby to sleep in a rocking chair. As the baby gets older, play routines with fathers are important developmentally. If feeding is very important to the father, he may feed the baby meals whenever he is there, once other foods besides mother's milk are introduced.

Check with your birth attendant or childbirth education instructor if she or anyone else is offering classes for new parents. The new trend among childbirth educators is new parent education classes, usually a series of meetings for the graduates of the Lamaze or Bradley course after the baby has been born. This new kind of class, in addition to expanding upon the parent education offered in high school health education courses, will begin to fill a void for new parents that has existed for more than 100 years, since the dissolution of the extended family. Present society does not give enough support to the full-time job of parenting. As you and the baby's father struggle along, sometimes without any support at all, you can be confident that in spite of the mistakes you may be making, the love will come through.

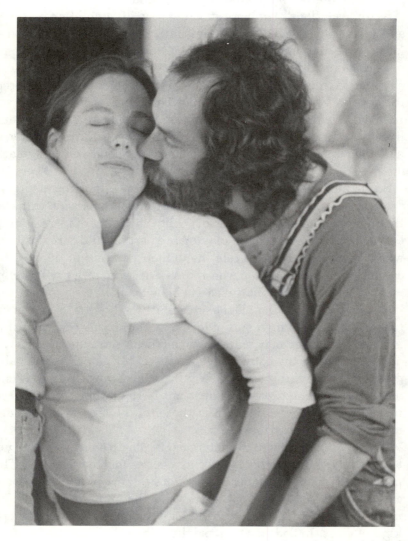

Byron Greatorex photograph

CHAPTER 9

If Hospital Birth Is Required

Hospitalization in and of itself is an intervention in the normal process of labor and delivery. For one thing, hospitals are dangerous. According to a 1986 newsletter of the Health Alternatives Legal Foundation, the Centers for Disease Control in Atlanta report that each year approximately two million patients pick up an infection in the hospital that they didn't have when they arrived, and more than 20,000 of these patients die as a direct or indirect result of such infections.[1]

Nevertheless, some people require hospital birth. Perhaps you have been planning a home birth but you learn you are expecting twins or your baby is in a breech position or you become ill. You and your birth attendant agree that these are factors which make home birth too risky for you. Or maybe you can't find a home birth attendant at all. Or, for whatever reason, maybe you just aren't ready to have a home birth.

CONTINGENCY PLANS

Even if none of the above applies to you, you will still want to have a contingency plan worked out on the chance that hospitalization becomes necessary. It is much easier to proceed with a clear mind about a home birth if you know you have good hospital backup. "Good" means not only that you have worked out a plan for getting to the hospital and that a doctor of your choice will meet you there, but also that the particular doctor and hospital agree on your requirements for birth.

Couples who have planned on home birth and who then must be hospitalized for birth feel disappointed and sad. Their midwife and other support people will be called upon to help them work out their feelings. Remember that although a hospital can never duplicate the home, no matter how colorfully the labor room is decorated, many of the advantages of the home can still be brought to the hospital. Even at home, couples may find that something they had hoped to do is impossible because the course of labor and birth are not predictable. The ideal home birth may be just a goal. So you must take steps beforehand to insure that no matter where birth takes place it is as near as possible to how you want it to be.

Several variables contribute to how well you plan a hospital birth. Some of them are: whether you have a doctor giving you prenatal care who knows about your home birth plans and shares your philosophy about making a hospital birth as homelike as possible; whether the hospital(s) available to you in your area already have homelike facilities, or if not, how much change from current hospital procedures you may be able to expect before your due date; and whether, if you are surely planning on home birth, you feel it is a waste of your time or psychologically demoralizing to plan actively the details of hospitalization.

Priorities for a Good Birth

The suggestions given apply to someone who is likely to have a hospital birth, because most require the time and ability to seek out facilities which offer these services. But your feelings on hospital birth should be discussed fully with your husband and your prospective birth attendant anyway, so that if you are planning a home birth but end up in the emergency room of a strange hospital, your support people can help you achieve the most important of your goals. It is a good idea to make a mental or written list of your priorities. You may not feel so strongly about enemas but may refuse to be attached to a fetal monitor without a medical reason or absolutely refuse to give up your healthy baby to a central nursery. If your hospitalization is unexpected, you may not even bother to mention your aversion to an enema or a shave since these things may seem unimportant compared to your emergency situation, and, in a hospital, you can't expect to fight and win about everything. But if your hospitalization is planned, a less important procedure may be a bargaining point on which you "give in" in exchange for avoiding a procedure you feel is even more potentially dangerous to you or your new baby's well-being.

HOW TO GET THE BEST FROM A HOSPITAL

There are several points to know about your rights and hospitalization. The American Hospital Association has adopted a Patient's Bill of Rights which it makes available to hospitals.[2] This bill of rights is not binding on a hospital, so it may have been rejected entirely, or a copy may be posted in the admitting office or a revised copy as it applies to that particular hospital may actually be handed to you. From a consumer point of view the AHA Bill of Rights still leaves things to be desired. But it does show that even hospitals will agree that you have the right to refuse procedures if you wish.

You should also know that you do have other rights even if they are not written in a patient's bill of rights. There is no law that says you must give up your civil rights or human rights just because you enter a hospital. George Annas, a lawyer, points out that if a hospital detains you at the scheduled release time because of nonpayment of a bill, you may sue it for false imprisonment.[3] Stating your intent to do so will probably ensure a speedy release. Another good point to know concerning leaving the hospital is that if you and your baby leave earlier than the time the hospital is willing to discharge you, you are not required by law to sign a release form.

A good general rule for trying to get what you want when you are up against established authority is to speak intelligently in an organized, pleasant way, trying not to raise your voice. Although when you are very emotionally involved, it may be difficult not to cry or act hysterical in the hospital, such emotional displays may work against you. In one case where crying worked, a mother hospitalized for surgery tried to convince the doctors to allow her husband to bring their nursing baby to visit her. Appeals about keeping her milk supply going, avoiding infection due to plugged milk ducts, and improving patient care by keeping morale high caused no result. But after an unexpected visit from a doctor who found the mother distraught and crying uncontrollably, he told her, "I didn't know you felt so deeply about this," and arranged to have her husband bring the baby. In another case, however, a frequently crying mother was distressed over the separation caused by her baby remaining in the central nursery. She was told she was "hysterical," practically forced to take a sedative by injection against her wishes, visited by four psychiatrists, and thereafter treated coldly.

In order to appear calm and reasonable it may be a good idea in the months preceding birth to anticipate what you will say in the expected situations. One general attitude to follow is: "I will let you do this if you can give me a good medical reason." Answers that amount to "This is always done" or "hospital policy" are not good medical reasons if they don't apply to you or your baby as individuals. Another good question is: "Can you guarantee the safety of this procedure?" A doctor could not honestly answer yes to this question for most procedures, from administering drugs to you in labor to giving the new baby sugar water. Once safety cannot be guaranteed, you have a quick way of sensibly explaining why you cannot permit what you don't want.

If you are hospitalized, it is probably because you and your doctor agree that there is good reason to be so. If you respect your doctor's judgment, certain medical procedures must be accepted, possibly without your fully understanding them, in a life-threatening situation. For example, there may not be adequate time for you to weigh the risks of continuing a very long labor when the electronic fetal monitor is showing "fetal distress" against the risks of major surgery in the immediate cesarean that the doctor is suggesting. But there may be time to request a blood sample from the baby's scalp to see if a low pH. will confirm oxygen deprivation.

Participation in decisions like this is an important part of your childbirth rights. These rights will be challenged constantly by hospital personnel who feel that such participation interferes with their job. You have the right to know the name and position of all hospital employees who enter the room, their purpose there, whether what they advise you to do has potential harm to you or your baby, and what alternatives are available. This information should be forthcoming from the employee as part of the doctrine of informed consent, and you should not be made to feel like an ornery patient if you have to request it.

It is also helpful to know that other major organizations support many of the points that parents make when they are negotiating their rights for hospital birth. For example, you may want to request the "Summary Report" of the Joint Interregional Conference on Appropriate Technology for Birth which was sponsored by the World Health Organization of the United Nations in April 1985.[4] At this conference, attended by over sixty participants from North and South America and Europe, some general recommendations included statements such as: "Clearly, there is no justification in any specific geographic region to have more than 10–15 percent cesarean section births" and "There is no evidence that routine intrapartum electronic fetal monitoring has a positive effect on the outcome of pregnancy." It also may be useful to read and quote from both the "Standards for Obstetric-Gynecologic Services" from the American College of Obstetricians and Gynecologists and the "Standards and Recommendations for Hospital Care of Newborn Infants" from the American Academy of Pediatrics because they contain statements which confirm your way of thinking.[5] It is a good idea to point out when a change proposed by you is not prohibited by state law. Even hospital administrators sometimes mistakenly act as if there were a divine law against practices such as allowing siblings in the delivery room. If you and your childbirth instructor are willing, you may want to arrange for a meeting with someone at the hospital, where she or he can present written medical evidence and you can explain from a personal consumer point of view what services you would be interested in and how they would benefit your family. Make sure that the hospital official you deal with puts in writing whatever accommodations are made for you that differ from the usual policy. This will avoid a lot of unnecessary grief for you if you enter the hospital at night when the administrator is home sleeping and the nurse on duty doesn't believe you.

WRITTEN BIRTH PLANS

One way that some parents protect themselves in hospital birth is by preparing a written birth plan. This plan can be discussed with the doctor ahead of time and then stapled to your chart in the office file and on your reservation when it is sent ahead to the hospital. If an item on the birth plan requires a major departure from hospital policy, it may be a good idea to get a copy of a letter from a hospital administrator giving permission for you to practice your option if there are no medical contraindications. Copies of this could also be made available along with the birth plan. Copies of the birth plan and any letters should also be brought by the couple to the hospital when the mother is admitted in case the ones attached to the chart are "lost." The birth plan could be both part of a hospital back-up plan for a home birth couple or part of the scheduled plan if hospital birth is definite.

Following is an example of one mother's birth plan. It is being presented because it is diplomatically yet forcefully phrased and because it covers many topics—not because you will necessarily agree with all the mother's choices. But it may be a good starting point for your own birth plan.

The mother called the plan "Requests for Our Child's Birth," and first listed the names of the hospital, the parents, the midwives, the obstetrician, the pediatrician, and the approximate delivery date. Then she wrote the following introduction:

> Because it is difficult to hold discussions and make decisions during the involvement of labor and delivery, we here express well in advance our concerns and expectations for this very special experience in our lives as individuals and as a family. We expect to rely on the normal physiological processes of labor and delivery to the maximum extent possible. By having routine interventions withheld and insuring as far as possible a natural family-centered birth, we feel the healthiest, least complicated and most satisfying birth experience is, in fact, most likely to happen.
>
> We, the parents, realize flexibility and a willingness to accept change in our plan may be necessary. In the event of complications or medical emergency, we will cooperatively confer with our midwives and our obstetrician whose judgment we respect and trust. Our participation in all aspects of the birth is very important to us.
>
> We hope the following requests will be respected to the fullest extent possible.

Now, the actual plan. (The rationale behind some of the mother's requests is given in brackets after that request.)

LABOR

Clinical admission by midwife

Husband remain with mother without separation

Assistance of midwife and childbirth educator [this mother had a labor coach in addition to her husband], as needed throughout labor
Hospital personnel respect the total privacy of mother, father, midwife, and labor coach
No set time limits for first and second stage [the mother means actual labor as "first stage" and the expulsion of the baby as "second stage"]
Suspension of routine medical procedures

- no prep or enema
- no electronic fetal monitor; request full reliance on fetal stethoscope
- no artificial rupture of membranes
- no IV; request fluids and light eating as desired by mother for hydration and energy. If IV becomes medically necessary, request it be placed high on mobile stand
- no sedatives, tranquilizers, analgesics, anesthesia
- no labor stimulants

Minimum of internal exams [the mother felt that the more she was examined, the more the chance of infection increased]
Use of bathroom encouraged; shower as needed
Mobility unrestricted and encouraged; no routine confinement to bed or labor room [it is important not to confine *yourself* to a specific position for labor, but merely to guarantee yourself *flexibility*]
Mother's own clothing from home, if she desires
Use of personal possessions such as radio, camera, toothbrush, pillows, mat, mirror, powder

DELIVERY

Delivery in labor room
Husband present at all times
Nonlithotomy position: flexibility of delivery position and freedom of movement; no straps and no stirrups
Spontaneous delivery as far as possible
Full information and informed consent at the time for medications, instrumentation, or anesthesia should they become medically necessary
No routine episiotomy; prefer massage with vitamin E oil, warm compresses, slower delivery with baby panted out and support to perineum
Mother able to touch baby's head and help deliver her baby if she desires; mirror available, no draping
Father may help deliver baby, if he desires [this is an example of how parents sometimes put things in birth plans that, in negotiations, they will "throw away" in deference to the doctor; the mother actually knew that the father had no interest in catching the baby]
After cord stops pulsating, father may cut cord
Presence of baby's sibling if he is accompanied by a responsible adult and if parents and sibling desire it

Spontaneous delivery of placenta; no uterine stimulants
Parents bathe baby
No recovery room

BABY AND AFTERBIRTH

Immediate and sustained contact with parents; baby placed on mother's abdomen
Immediate breastfeeding
Delay of eyedrops and of nonlifesaving routines (e.g., weighing, measurements, footprinting) until after bonding
Suctioning of baby only as needed
Use of erythromycin; no silver nitrate
If baby showing no signs of distress, baby warmed by mother's body
Vernix rubbed into baby
Baby stays with mother and father at all times
Baby care, including pediatrician's exam, in presence of mother and father

- baby not taken to nursery
- if nursery a necessity, baby accompanied by parent(s) and stays there as short a time as possible

Baby examined by our appointed private pediatrician or house resident immediately after birth
Only essential tests performed
Sibling be allowed to meet and enjoy baby with parents as soon as possible after birth if he has not already witnessed birth
No circumcision in hospital
24-hour rooming-in, beginning immediately
Discharge mother and baby from hospital as soon as desired (within eight hours)
Baby totally breastfed; no bottles

IF CESAREAN DELIVERY BECOMES NECESSARY

That the decision be a cooperative one between parents, midwife, and obstetrician
That parents be informed at all times of events and advised of all possible choices and outcomes before consent is given
Husband present at all times during cesarean (regional or general anesthesia), including for administration of anesthesia
That decision regarding type of anesthesia (spinal, epidural, or general) and preoperative and postoperative medications be a cooperative one between doctors and parents
Mother to be awake throughout entire procedure, including repair, if possible
No obstruction of mother's view; lower screen during procedure or use mirror
One hand free to permit immediate breastfeeding, holding, and bonding after delivery

After birth that baby, if stable and not in distress, also be given to father to hold for extended time

Request ongoing commentary of procedure from surgeon, anesthesiologist, or surgical nurse during surgery

Father and baby allowed to stay with mother during repair

Father with mother in recovery room

Special care nursery only if absolutely necessary

24-hour rooming-in begun as soon as possible

Mother be allowed a 24-hour helper (husband and/or relative)

Postoperative medications only as needed and requested

EMERGENCY and/or LIFE-THREATENING SITUATIONS
If baby requires Intensive Care Unit

- father goes with baby
- baby receives mother's pumped breast milk and begin breastfeeding as soon as possible
- if baby must be transferred to another hospital, family goes as a unit

If complications arise at birth

- father not asked to leave at any time
- coach/midwife present at all times
- all previous requests honored to extent possible

If labor difficult or emergency procedure becomes necessary, sibling be permitted (accompanied by an adult) to join with parents and new baby as soon as mother and baby are in recovery, if so desired

If death of either mother or baby anticipated, all family members (parents and sibling) be together

If baby dies, that parents be given time together to see and hold baby and that baby remain property of family to plan family grieving

It would be a good idea if your doctor initials whatever your plan provides before having it stapled to your office and hospital charts.

Many parents include in their birth plans a stipulation about leaving the hospital earlier than the usual stay, if the mother and baby are in good health. But you should be prepared for what happens at some hospitals when you make your wishes known. Medical personnel will imply or state outright that you risk bringing your baby back Dead-on-Arrival and in general express a "don't-call-us-when-you-start-to-hemorrhage" attitude. You are not legally bound to sign forms absolving the hospital of responsibility, but it might be the only convenient way to get your baby out of the nursery. If no one has given you a satisfactory medical reason why you or your baby requires further hospitalization, you are probably correct in following your own feelings about early discharge. Most people rest, recuperate, and care for their new baby better under the loving guidance of their families on their own familiar turf. A few health insurance carriers now encourage early discharge and will pay for a visiting nurse or other caregiver to come to the home.

Even if complications require your having a cesarean, the experience does not have to be totally without loving support. More hospitals now permit fathers in the operating room for cesareans, and the mother can receive a local anesthetic so she, too, can share the excitement of birth. If you have already had a cesarean operation, you probably will not try to have a home birth, although many women have been successful at this. The risk of rupture of the uterine scar from the previous cesarean is so small that most "home VBACs" (vaginal birth after cesarean) are successful. Certainly if you are planning a hospital VBAC you should shop around for an obstetrician who has a good reputation for success. The ACOG now recommends VBAC in many cases.

CONSUMERISM

Hospitals make changes in their procedure—husband in the delivery room, to use the most widespread example—almost exclusively because of consumer pressure. Few doctors have ever welcomed incursions onto their territory; policies change when the hospital begins to lose money. To put it another way, if you had two hospitals in your community and one offered family-centered maternity care and one didn't, which hospital would you use?

So, if you have contacted more than one hospital, make sure you tell the ones you don't choose why they weren't chosen. Then they will understand that they have lost thousands of dollars because you are going to a better hospital. Because of factors ranging from a slowing birth rate to a growing home birth movement, hospitals often operate their maternity wings at a loss. If they lose more and more money, they will eventually end their maternity services, unless they respond to consumer demand to revamp their services.

An alternative to both hospital and home birth is the maternity home. The concept is popular in a number of other countries but hardly recognized in the United States. The best known here is the Maternity Center Association's Childbearing Center in New York City. There, carefully selected couples give birth in a cheerful labor-delivery area in a refurbished brownstone, attended by a nurse-midwife. The parents hold and love their baby for twelve hours before medical checkups and discharge. There is oxygen available, but no facilities for surgery; a waiting ambulance connects to a hospital eleven minutes away. Center personnel hope to draw back into the system couples who would otherwise have an unattended home birth. Yet for many couples, weighing the increased inconvenience, foreign germs, and less familiar surroundings, the home still wins out, since their apartment in New York City is usually no more than eleven minutes from the closest hospital also. Other couples who reject hospitalization are forced into a home birth by the Childbearing Center's strict standards. These include, among others, not accepting a couple into the program once the fetus is past twenty-four weeks' gestation. But rigid standards will help keep the Childbearing Center's statistics nearly perfect, which is what is needed to convince some still skeptical doctors in the community. For couples who reject the hospital but reject home birth, too, the Childbearing Center is the perfect answer. What is most important is that the woman have choices and the cooperation of trained personnel, whether the choice of birth site is the home, maternity center, or hospital.

Consumers can continue to look forward to new alternatives like these in response to their requirements, whether the motivation of doctors and hospitals is financial, which it often is, or deep concern for respecting the needs of patients. Where there is mutual respect and cooperation between health care providers and consumers, a mutually agreeable solution can be found.

Still, no matter how many temporary victories are scored for the human rights of hospital patients, it is difficult to be totally satisfied with institutional birth. At any rate, if you have to go to the hospital, you have to go to the hospital. Tell yourself that, in the end, no mater what happens, you will soon get back home and do it *your* way.

CHAPTER 10

Dealing with the World

In September 1987 a mother from Massachusetts sat on the stage on Phil Donohue's television talk show and told millions of people how the Department of Social Services accused her of sexually abusing her children because she let her young daughters sleep in her bed, and the four-year-old still breastfed.

Ten years earlier a New York mother had been banned from her village pool because she discreetly nursed her baby at the toddler pool while minding her two older children. And a year later an Iowa firefighter who had been nursing her baby daughter at the fire house during her personal time required a court hearing and an investigation by the Iowa Civil Rights Commission to determine that she really had that right.

While the daily experiences of most of us don't make the headlines, people like the complaining neighbors in Massachusetts, New York, and Iowa live all around us. Having your baby at home and then raising that baby in the way outlined here will almost surely subject you to some kind of harassment from relatives, doctors, neighbors, friends, and acquaintances; it may be very subtle but strike you very deeply. Coping with others' attitudes is a some-times-neglected topic but one which must be dealt with realistically. Depending on the type of feedback you get and the type of person you are, you will probably need varying degrees of support during your pregnancy and after your baby is born at home. These supports may range from sharing your daily experiences with your mate as a way of giving vent to your emotions to attempting to limit your daily encounters almost exclusively to those people who agree with you. This will not be easy if you live in an isolated area where you have little choice of acquaintances and medical services.

DISAPPROVAL

Being a nonconformist has never been easy. If you do things like having your baby at home, breastfeeding past a year (the American Academy of Pediatrics now recommends breastfeeding for a year), or allowing your son to play with a doll, you may experience occurrences like the following, which all have really happened to mothers:

- You excitedly but carefully explain to your gynecologist, whom you regard as your long-standing personal physician since he has treated you for years for more than just vaginal infections, that you would like to have the baby at home. This doctor, who has never spent more than five minutes of discussion time with you after an examination, spends twenty minutes yelling at you, berating you, calling your idea "frankly the dumbest thing I've ever heard," citing horrendous birth tales he has witnessed, including genetically malformed babies, and concluding by instructing you never to come back to his office again until you get "such a stupid idea" out of your head.
- Your husband's aunt asks you, in front of the two of you, if it's true you didn't have an episiotomy. When you say it is true, she says to you, with a rather questioning look at your husband, "Well, you must be very big." You recall the scene in a funny book you once read where a woman sitting on a soda fountain stool suddenly sinks down because her vagina is so big, as you realize your aunt is feeling very sorry for her nephew and the awful sex life he must have.
- Your neighbor comments, with an odd smile, that the doll you bought your son for Christmas must be the reason he appears to act "like a mother" (meaning nicely) to the new baby.

- Your child's pediatrician asks you in an exasperated tone why you are "making it very difficult" for him. You are aware that you have been unable to answer in a specific way most of his questions. These have included: "How many times a day does the baby nurse?" (Answer: "I never counted. Whenever he seems to want to.") "How many times a day does the baby nap?" (Answer: same as before) "How long does he breastfeed on each side?" (Answer: "Well, it varies.") "How often does the baby wake at night?" (Answer: same as before, or, if you really have nerve and with an embarrassed laugh: "Well, you know, I just take him in with me so each time he wakes I don't turn on the lights and look at the clock and maybe I just switch him to the other breast and doze off again. . . . ")
- Your mother calls repeatedly and asks, "How is it I never hear the baby cry?" You feel like saying, "Because I am doing such a good job," while you know she is thinking, "I wonder what's wrong with the baby?" (You will learn to accept comments on how little the baby cries and how content the baby seems at adult parties as the only compliments you may get.)
- An old friend tells you she is sorry she has to ask you this, but please don't breastfeed the baby "in public" the next time she and her family visit your home. She explains that her growing daughter is at "that impressionable age when you have to be careful what she's exposed to."

If tales like these, which are not uncommon, occur to you several times in one day or week, you may find yourself reduced to tears and depression. It is difficult to feel as if you are the only one who does things your way. The knowledge that you are not alone doesn't always help, because the closest mother who thinks like you may live in another community and you may never meet her. There is inner torment in feeling like that lone soldier who marched the opposite way. We live in a world where many people don't even know the name of the drug they are taking and where many never question if it has side-effects to their bodies. You are taking on a big responsibility in your family, in your circle of friends, and in your community if you are the first to question standard medical practice by going against the advice of your doctor and, perhaps equally as serious for you, the advice of your mother and your mother-in-law.

You will first become aware of the strong feeling of others against your way of doing things when you are pregnant. The initial concern of close family members, besides that you are gaining too much weight, is that your plans for home birth are risky. You may admit that there is some element of risk in a home birth, just as there is some risk in everything one does, but that you are doing everything you can to prevent or predict any risk. You may explain that if your pregnancy is normal and you are healthy, there may be more risk to hospital birth for you. This is something your family will find hard to believe, but it is worth repeating many times with proof. Hart Collins, a home birth mother, finally came to realize, "The hospital was merely an excuse, it seemed, to pin the guilty label on someone else for an unhappy experience."

Unfortunately, you may have a hard time finding a sympathetic listener for your concerns about the birth—not specifically home birth. Most women don't express the common fear of having a malformed or sick baby, but if you do mention it, or if you voice other normal concerns such as your insecurity over impending first-time motherhood, a home birth adversary will be quick to insist that hospitalization would be the best way to "solve" any problems.

The worst victims of society's attitudes are those few couples who do experience problems with the birth. If a woman hemorrhages after a home birth, is taken to the hospital, treated, and released, some families seem more intent on harboring an "I told you so" attitude than on being relieved at the happy outcome. The reaction is stronger still if the baby is the one with the problem. In one instance a home born baby cried almost constantly and could rarely be calmed. The parents brought the baby to the hospital the next morning, where he died of a congenital heart defect. Although the hospital doctor told the parents that the defect was so severe that the baby could not have been saved in any case, the county coroner visited the parents at home, questioned them extensively, and clearly implied they had killed their child through neglect. This family had also lost a child they had never seen or held after a hospital birth, and the mother expressed gratitude that the home born baby had at least known their love before he died. Anthropologist Lester Hazell has aptly noted, in *Commonsense Childbirth,* "If anything goes wrong you are in a position of having brought it on yourself and your baby. Our strange society will not hold it against you if your baby is palsied or has his intelligence stunted by too much anesthesia in the hospital, but if he is born at home with a birthmark or a clubfoot, the fault will be called yours."

This kind of attitude may be expected, and many home birth couples are prepared for it. They have already decided that they will not change their plans unless there is a good medical reason to do so. Knowing the relationships you have with your friends and family members, you will choose whom you will turn a deaf ear to and whom you will painstakingly try to convince to accept your decision.

What you are not prepared for probably is the attitude of family, friends, and the medical profession *after* the baby is born and both mother and child are fine. For the woman intent on practicing natural mothering, the oppression doesn't end at birth but only grows with the child.

Medical Interference

The offenders with the most damaging influence are in the medical profession. Many doctors recommend unnecessary and possibly harmful practices which interfere with successful lactation. Among these are frequent washing of the nipples (which can actually cause soreness), early introduction of supplements to a healthy baby (which can actually spur allergies and digestive upsets), and early and abrupt weaning (which can cause trauma to mother and child if neither wanted to wean). A rather common difficulty is an infected milk duct, for which frequent nursing, not weaning, is the best cure and the best preventative of further backup and infection. If an antibiotic is prescribed, this is also not usually cause for even temporary cessation of breastfeeding.

Most doctors just do not appear to realize how much nursing means to the mother. If the doctor feels certain that temporary weaning is a medical necessity, which is rare, he should work with the mother to see that the nursing relationship can be resumed as soon as possible. Many mothers mistakenly assume that their doctors are sympathetic, since most say they are in favor of breastfeeding. But for nonmedical questions, the doctor's answers may be just another parent's opinions, to be given no more weight than advice from a neighbor on how she puts her children to bed.

The lack of understanding by professionals of the strong ties mothers feel for their babies may lead to further abuse of the mother. The example of the mother from Massachusetts is a case in point. Although we might be shocked by the idea of a four-year-old at the breast, we can think back to many children we know who were attached to their bottles past the age of three. Apparently our society sees this as "normal" while a mother nursing an older child is often regarded as "sick"—although bottlefeeding was originally designed as a substitute for and imitation of breastfeeding.

In addition to breastfeeding beyond a year, bringing the baby to bed with you is another subject where a nearly universal negative reaction is encountered in doctors, family, and friends. The practice is common in nearly every other country in the world; it is a great convenience for night feedings, and it is a great comfort to a little baby. Yet the reaction from nearly everyone you respect or love is usually disgust. The way in which this reaction is expressed may strike you like a physical blow. This is another area where it cannot be repeated often enough that *you* are the parents of your baby and that *you* are the ones best equipped with the knowledge and feelings to decide what is best. It sometimes seems that other people are saying that things which make you and the baby unhappy, such as the infant crying, are good ("It's good for his lungs; let him cry it out") while things which make you and the baby happy, such as a contented breastfeeding, are bad ("Look how you both enjoy it; he'll get spoiled.") Wouldn't it seem that if these people also cared about the best interests of you and your baby, they would be happy when you and your baby are happy, sad when you are both sad?

Doctors, relatives, and friends will also be frequently concerned about whether the baby is sleeping through the night (which realistically may not happen for a very long time) and in general whether your baby is "good" (is a baby crying in a crib for thirty minutes an indication of a bad baby or a bad mother?). You will also be encouraged to leave the baby and go out, even if you don't want to leave your baby when she is very young; if you refuse to go out or decide to take the baby with you, you will be criticized for having a baby who "rules your life." You may be ashamed to admit it if you like being a mother or ashamed that the attitude of your parents has caused you to wonder what kind of parents they were if they appear to be so unwilling to give of themselves to another little person. In sum, although you may have started out feeling that your ideas on childbirth and childrearing were indicators of your desire to give your child the best start possible in life, the constant comments of relatives, friends, and doctors seem to indicate that you are doing the worst job possible.

COPING

It is no wonder then that a large number of home birth parents find they must retreat into silence or lies after the baby is born. They learn they cannot even share photos of the birth with some people who are close to them. Being devoted parents with strong feelings of love for the baby appears to some as aberrant behavior. Trusting your own feelings is somehow not scientific enough. (We all enjoyed the research study, which was reported in *Psychology Today* and *Parents* in 1986, that the more you carry a baby around, the less she or he will cry.) It may be that you cannot talk about your childbearing and childrearing beliefs to many people. This may hurt you, because during the early weeks and months especially you may have negative and conflicting feelings about the demands of parenthood and may want to share them with people close to you. During this time you may often feel discouraged and tired. You have little perspective. It seems as if the intensity of the moment is endless. It may take two full months before you can let the baby sleep a long time without feeling his back to check on breathing. A diaper rash may seem like a personal failing, and you pray for the passage of time when the "tragedy" will be over. You may also have an image of what the perfect mother is like— clean home, contented baby, happy husband, svelte figure, working and nursing and socializing all at once—and you always seem far from the ideal, although you know that no one is the mother in the television commercials. Unfortunately, this is another time when some relatives may respond with "I told you so," if you share these feelings. It will be helpful to share your negative as well as positive thoughts with your husband, or try to find another supportive mother.

It is not easy to learn what is bothering many of your relatives, friends, and acqaintances. Perhaps they are jealous that you and your child are having an opportunity they will never have. More than likely, your way of doing things is a challenge to how they have borne and raised children. They have always thought of their way of scheduling and tidiness as the "right" way. Your parents may feel that your way is a blatant rejection of how they parented you. After all, if you were satisfied with their way, why would you do it another way? They may act as if you are just rebelling, not realizing that your ideas are based on careful research and thought, and this may further hurt you because it does not show you the respect you deserve. What your parents and you must realize is that there are no guarantees for any way of bringing up children. There are many factors that are beyond the control of two parents. But you are choosing what seems the best way for you and your child, to the best of your control, knowledge, and feelings, just as your parents made what were the best decisions to them when you were born. You are now an equal parent with the right to make good decisions, and some mistakes, too. Once it was their turn, and now it is yours. Good parents should support you, not just condemn you, as you now grope your way through parenthood.

You will be lucky if during this period someone will "mother" you, too. After the birth, which is a time of elation, there occurs a "coming down" period when the new family must again deal with the ordinary world. Going from a "high" to normality may be depressing in itself. And you will have to deal with other concerns as well. Many of your deep-seated fears about blood and death, your own feelings about breasts and sexuality, and your resolution of feminist issues may have all come to the fore during pregnancy, childbirth, and child care.

To set your course straight again you may often want to remind yourself of the answer to the important question: "What is the job of a parent?" You are nurturing your child, meeting her needs as fully as possible, knowing that all the love and security you give now will make you child feel good and be better able to cope with the world when the time for letting go is at hand. To be there when your child needs you is and always will be your job as a parent. It is important to persevere: it is your body, your baby, your life. Trust yourself to do what you know is best.

CHAPTER 11

Family Stories

1. ON THE EIGHTH FLOOR OF AN APARTMENT BUILDING ON NEW YORK'S WEST SIDE

L aura, an artist, was in her late twenties and had been married for six years when she and her husband Duval, a lawyer, decided to try to have a baby. Laura had just stopped taking birth control pills after long-term usage, and there was difficulty conceiving. So after about a year and a half of trying, Laura and Duval went to see an obstetrician/gynecologist who was known as a fertility expert. Laura was actually pregnant during her first visit to his office, although she didn't realize it at the time.

Early in the pregnancy Laura and Duval also went to another obstetrician who was connected with a health insurance plan they subscribed to. Although Laura liked this woman, the couple decided to go back to the fertility expert because, they were advised, he was known as an expert and he was with a well-known university hospital.

"It's funny how much you repress at the time," Laura recalls.

"You take the doctor's advice without questioning it. When I look back on it now, I realize how brusque he was."

Laura's pregnancy was normal. Regarding nutrition, her doctor's advice was to take one prenatal tablet a day and not to gain more than twelve to fifteen pounds. Laura says she knew "twenty to twenty-five pounds was sort of typical," but she just told herself, " 'Oh, well, I guess he thinks I'm a little overweight to begin with' and I didn't think too much of it. I ended up gaining twenty-five pounds anyway, in spite of him."

Laura and Duval took the childbirth preparation course at the hospital. "And this I think was one of the factors that upset me the most," Laura says. "We were prepared for a natural delivery—films, breathing, etc." Laura's labor began with contractions at about three in the morning, and she went into the hospital at around ten. Laura remembers the doctor telling her that the baby was in a posterior position, "and because of the posterior position and first pregnancy, he expected a long, sort of drawn out labor. Therefore, he advised that I have *Pitocin,* which would speed up the labor, right? Ignoramus that I was, I had an IV, and I had a partial prep, and I had an enema, and all those terrible things. Oh, and he broke the bag of water."

Laura says that the early part of her labor was rather pleasant; it was in the daytime and everyone appeared to be in good spirits. Laura was knitting and her husband and doctor were reading the *New York Times.*

"But I remember when the *Pitocin* took effect, it was as though I was totally out of control. I really could barely stay on top of the contractions. I remember looking at the doctor desperately and saying, 'Just what do I do,' in terms of breathing. And he said, 'Do whatever you feel necessary,' which I did. He turned the infant around in utero, which—it wasn't painful but it was incredibly uncomfortable and a very strange sensation. Anyway, the time came when he said, 'Push! Push!' And I had absolutely no urge to push. No sensation.

"Then he said something about, 'We've got to get her to the delivery room right now,' you know, there's fetal distress. So they whipped me into the delivery room and knocked me out with what-ever it was, nitrous oxide I guess, and did an episiotomy and a forceps delivery. And she was fine, I guess. They told me everything was okay.

"But I can remember, oh, when I was taken back into the labor room, they told me that it was 'changing of the guard' for the nurses and that I couldn't go down to my room on the floor where the babies were for a few hours. And I remember crying immediately after the birth because first of all I felt I had failed. I had been totally prepared for something that didn't happen the way I expected it. And I couldn't see my baby.

"At the time I felt, 'Well, he did the best he could, and I'm glad he saved her from whatever distress she was experiencing.' And yet I recall being just so sad, as though the one thing I really felt I could do on my own, deliver my own child, had been taken away from me.

"Looking back, I have negative feelings. Things keep coming to mind, even years later. After reading *Immaculate Deception,* I remember I said to Duval, 'My goodness! I've repressed so much.' All these negative feelings that were, at the time, just a kind of hurt, a sadness. The nighttime feedings, for example. I remember it very distinctly, expecting my child to be brought to me for nursing when she was hungry. Whenever she was brought to me in the evening, she had this sort of weird, spaced-out look, as though she had been crying for a while, until they finally brought her to me. I do remember one night waking up and going to the bathroom, and looking into the nursery, and seeing her crying there. She had been taken aside, and there was a bottle on a table, but there was no nurse in sight. The nurse had obviously been giving her a bottle and had left for some reason. And here was this kid crying. I got the feeling that the nurses acted like robots. They treated and handled so many thousands of babies, they really didn't care."

When baby Hilary was about eighteen months old the family moved to Boston for two years. At about the time they were contemplating a second child, a friend of theirs there had her second child at home, and "It started me thinking about home delivery," Laura says. "She said it's so nice to have everything relaxed and everybody around you acting normally."

Laura, Duval, and Hilary moved back to New York. They decided definitely to have another baby. The obstetrician who had delivered Hilary had moved to Ohio. "Luckily, I feel now," says Laura, "because I probably would have just fallen back into the groove by going back to him. So I just let it lie for a while. Then a woman in our baby-sitting cooperative, who was pregnant, came over one night, and I asked, 'Who is your doctor? I'm going to need a doctor at some point.' And she hemmed and hawed and then said, 'Well, as a matter of fact, I don't have a doctor. I have a midwife, and I'm going to have a home delivery.' And she said it in an embarrassed way, you know, like she wasn't quite sure how I would respond. Well, I was ecstatic. I said, 'I had no idea that this was even possible in New York, and I would love to do the same thing.' "

Laura made an appointment with the nurse-midwife her new friend recommended, and soon after the first visit discovered she was pregnant. Prenatal examinations were done either in Laura's or the midwife's nearby apartment. "The whole thing was so relaxed and peaceful," Laura says. "It was like having a visit with a friend. She'd stay a couple of hours and talk to me. And I understood for the first time what the whole concept of developing a relationship with a midwife was all about. You seldom have a chance to develop that kind of relationship with an obstetrician, at least a male one."

Laura also was impressed with the midwife's attitude toward nutrition. "She said she really wasn't concerned about how much weight I gained, as long as I was eating the right things." The midwife suggested two books as guidelines, including one by Adelle Davis. "And then later on, when I was well into the prenatal checkups, she asked for three days' worth of my diet, so she could make certain it was adequate, and it was. What I find to be true with midwives in terms of checking out diet and vitamins, and so on, is that their information is far superior to what any obstetrician has provided me. It impressed me."

She also found it "remarkable" that during a prenatal visit her midwife said to her, "Here are your medical records.' I've never in my life had any doctor show me medical records, even when I requested them. And here she was saying, 'Here they are. You ought to look at them.' "

Laura's labor, like the last one, began at about three o'clock one morning. As the hours wore on, Laura told Duval it was all right to go to work, warning him, 'Be prepared to come home because I really think this is it.' Looking back, I'm not sure that was the wisest thing," Laura says, "because ultimately he didn't get home soon enough for my liking." Laura called the midwife, who arrived at around ten in the morning and, after reviewing the situation, said she would come back around one, since both women had some errands to attend to. While the midwife went her way, Laura and

Hilary went to the bank and did the shopping. "And looking back on it," says Laura, "I was probably already in very active labor. There I was walking around, and I sort of had to stop for a few moments every time I had a contraction."

On returning home Laura discovered that although she had practiced her breathing exercises with Hilary around, there was still some explaining to do. "She'd ask me a question, and I'd have to go into my breathing for a contraction or two, and she'd say, 'Why aren't you answering me? Answer me!' I had to explain to her again why I had to breathe that way, and she finally caught on after a few silences. And then as I lay around and started breathing more rapidly, she said, 'Don't breathe so fast.' It concerned her, I guess. But she was okay. As things got down to serious business, she stayed put, was just an observer."

The midwife came back and confirmed that Laura was in active labor. She also said that although she had been in the anterior position the week before, the start of labor found the baby in the posterior position. Laura says this did not frighten her, recalling her first posterior labor. "Looking back on my previous obstetrician's excuse about the whole business . . . after the fact, I was only more annoyed at him. It's funny, you know, this birth was like the first one to me because I was really feeling things as if they were going on the first time. And I remember in transition, I kept saying, 'I can't do it. I'm not on top of it. I'm out of control.' And my midwife and an apprentice she had brought with her kept saying to each other, 'Oh, she's really doing a good job. She's really on top of it.' That's all I needed to hear.

"But for the most part the midwife stayed in the background except when she was needed. During the pushing stage—that was totally new to me—for as I said I hadn't felt the urge with Hilary. Apparently I wasn't pushing in the right direction, it was so new. And nothing was happening. I felt like I wanted to push, and yet it didn't work even when I did. We tried all sorts of different positions. I tried squatting, I tried all fours—nothing seemed to happen. And though I wasn't particularly aware of the time, apparently thirty or forty minutes had passed without any real progress. And the midwife was getting concerned, although at the time I wasn't aware of all this, and she finally said, 'Well, why don't you go to the bathroom and try that.' So I did. And apparently that did the trick. The baby turned around. You know, all of a sudden

I got the direction of the whole thing. So I got back into bed and things really started happening then. And I can remember thinking, 'Wow, this is really what it's like.' It's so scary the first time with the pushing. Even though you're telling yourself what's going on and what's going to happen, until the moment of expulsion you really don't know. Unnerving.

"But then once the head started coming out, it was fantastic. You can look down and see this head coming out, it's just tremendous. Then when she was born, I was totally calm. She was pink as soon as she came out, which was to be expected from all my reading—but she didn't cry. So the midwife decided she had to use flicking fingers on the feet, and spanking the feet—she tried massage at first, but nothing got her to cry. Finally she did, but it was sort of through typical hospital methods. You could see her chest moving up and down. Later I read the Leboyer book and it made me really sorry, because I would have insisted even on giving the baby a few more moments or something. The midwife claimed that the real reason she was disturbed was that the muscle tone wasn't as good as she would like. Anyway, it was six o'clock in the evening which was really a beautiful time."

2. PITTSBURGH STORY

Kenly didn't start dating until she was eighteen, but once she did she began to think about marriage. She had certain ideas about what she wanted in a husband. "I really was interested in what I called 'The Three Ms': someone who had a tremendous mind, maturity, and money. And I got them all in Tom."

What else came with the package was one of Tom's prerequisites for marriage, expressed when he proposed: he wanted three children, and he wanted them born at home. "He knew what he wanted," Kenly recalls. "He just knew from reading and studying and looking into things."

The idea was novel to Kenly, who was in the process of a medical education, taking her bachelor of science degree in nursing at the University of Maryland. Even at school, her first introduction to birth was atypical. "I saw a movie of a birth in nursing school. There she was, she had a baby, got up off the table, took her baby, and walked back to her room. Now [in those years] that was new to nursing, it was really new."

Tom also had ideas on when their first baby was to be born. "We wanted a January baby because he said that was the most intelligent month," Kenly says. "Of course, Tom was born in January." So after marriage, Kenly's graduation, and Tom's return from Vietnam, the couple settled down in Pittsburgh and started their first child. The due date would be March, but Tom didn't mind. The difficult hurdle was not the due date but finding a birth attendant before it came around. "I called all over, asking, 'Does the doctor deliver naturally?' " Kenly says. "And the response was, 'Naturally the doctor delivers babies. He's an obstetrician. Didn't you call him?' So I kept reading, kept looking, I did find a midwife, a granny midwife, and she said, 'Call back when you're seven months.' And when I called back, in my seventh month, she said she wasn't going to renew her license."

Kenly was not receiving prenatal care, although she now says she feels it is important. "At the time, I figured, a baby was natural, it would come naturally. But I was reading constantly. I kept reading. And, of course, I was a nurse. That helped. I think that also scares you, because you know all the possible dangers. And I think it's just natural what a first-time mother goes through, 'I hope he's normal, I hope he's healthy, with all the pieces in place.' And so we explored the pros and cons. We knew it was our baby, we had planned it at home, conceived it at home, and we'd have it at home. A family relationship is what we really wanted. I called and got no response from the doctors. We did go and visit one whose response was, 'I've delivered many babies, and it's such pain, and you don't want to suffer like that.' At least he didn't charge us anything for the visit. And Tom was there with me throughout the search. Because, at that time, nine years ago, I was a little kid. I was scared to death. Not of having a baby, but just of opening up and communicating my needs. Nine years ago, talking in front of doctors or anyone, I did not have confidence. I've learned since then."

Nearly at the end of Kenly's pregnancy, Tom had another good idea. At a club he belonged to, he asked around and found out that some of the members had had their babies at home. A general practitioner was recommended, an appointment was made, and Kenly was examined. The GP agreed to attend the baby's birth. But there was one stipulation: Kenly and Tom lived about ninety minutes away from this doctor, so they would have to travel to a house nearer by to have their baby. An acquaintance graciously offered her home and agreed to pamper Kenly and the new baby for as many days as necessary. Although some of the advantages of home birth would be lost, others would remain. So Kenly and Tom agreed.

Kenly began her first labor with a "feeling." She says, "I can't tell you, there wasn't any pain or tremendous pressure, it's just a feeling." She had even told her sister on the phone that day, "Well, I think it's gonna be tonight for me." By dawn she and Tom were at Nancy's house, with the doctor arriving soon after. Kenly's smallest baby, Rachel, eight pounds, twelve ounces, and nineteen inches, arrived a few hours later.

Kenly doesn't remember the birth fondly, because of her relationship with the doctor. "When you're going through the transition and someone tells you hurry up and have this baby or I'm going to sit in an easy chair—by that time I was ready to go and kick her into an easy chair. But still she was there. If I had known her personality, if I had been stronger, I would have joked with her, because she really was a dedicated person. But I pushed too soon and pushed too hard with the baby. Also, I was too uptight with the doctor. She was making me tense. And I pushed and pushed. And I was exhausted. I was angry. I was angry at her, and I was angry at my husband. He was holding my hand, he was really good, but I wanted him to tell her to shut up, and I lacked the nerve. And a woman gets frustrated, or anyone gets frustrated when they keep it in. She did an episiotomy and the baby did come. I was exhausted. Then the problems came afterward, with the hemorrhoids and the constipation, which seems normal, but I think if people relax, it doesn't have to be that way. Some people adored that doctor. I couldn't stand her, but that's all I had at the time."

The same doctor was still all Kenly had when she became pregnant again two years later. She hoped it would be different this time because Kenly, Tom, and Rachel had moved closer to where the doctor lived and would be having the second baby in their own home. And it was different. "The nicest thing about it was that the doctor didn't arrive in time for the birth. It was beautiful. No worry about tension and complaining."

The second labor began again with a feeling. "I simply knew I was in labor. Nothing big or painful. I just knew something was going on. And I called a friend who was a nurse, who had been with other people who had had babies. And the whole experience was really good, you know, a nice relaxing atmosphere, the best kind there is. I told my husband he could try the doctor, but he couldn't get her. Wasn't that nice?

"And the birth was beautiful. I was on my side for a long time. It must have been two hours. Tom would rub my back. It felt great. As soon as he took his hand off I'd say, 'Rub me again. Don't take your hand away.' Just that security of having someone there. And suddenly I felt like I couldn't be on my side anymore. I didn't do any pushing. The baby felt like a little lemon, and then it felt like a grapefruit. And, I was embarrassed. I was afraid. I said to my friend, 'Oh, check and see if I've had a bowel movement,' not just for neatness, but I didn't want to get the baby dirty. I didn't want to mess the baby up. And my friend is a real diplomat and she said calmly, 'Oh, Kenly, don't worry about it. Tom, you better come here, 'cause here's the head.' And there was the head. And it just came out beautifully—the head and then the shoulders. The cord was around the neck, and Tom knew to pull it off her neck.

"And then she was there and kind of quiet. She didn't yell much at all, you know, scream and holler. And so we just put her on my tummy and I held her and let her relax there for about an hour and she was really a long, thin, little ugly-looking baby. After I read Leboyer's book, I realize the experience was really a lot like the one he describes, because the baby didn't make noise. As a matter of fact, there was even a moment when I was upset because she wasn't making noise, so I picked her up and looked at her and she let out an 'Ahhh.' It was just pleasant, it really was. That was the birth of Elizabeth. The doctor came about an hour later and cut the cord. She said if I didn't push my placenta out already she'd get it out, and thinking of her doing that, I gave a push and it came out."

Kenly and Tom had another baby, Ruth, a little over a year later, after a surprise pregnancy and a two-and-a-half-hour labor. This birth had the advantage of their finding a new doctor, but the disadvantage of having again to travel to someone else's house to have the baby. Kenly was the tenth woman to have her baby at the woman's house. She says, "They were very nice people, but to be honest with you, I was not as comfortable. It was just not the same as having it in your own home." For this birth, too, the doctor did not come in time. "It was nice. It was a nice birth in that sense, but I honestly would have liked just my husband and myself. Because I was in the woman's house I felt obliged to have her there observing my birth, which was important to her. She was telling me when to push, and I shouldn't have listened, but I was still not strong enough to speak up." Tom caught this baby, too.

Kenly says other people's "best response" to her babies was, "She's smiling!'" All her babies smiled regularly by age three weeks. Other people would insist, "You know, they're not supposed to smile until later."

The three birth experiences have taught her, Kenly says, "to keep it in your own home with someone whom you really want there, whom you know, and if it is a doctor, you really have to talk it out beforehand. It depends on what people want. If they want the doctor there just to observe in case something goes wrong but they want the husband to deliver the baby—it's really what the doctor feels good with and the people feel good with. And I don't really feel you have to push. I feel that the babies will come out naturally, all by themselves. You don't have to sit there and say, "Wait. Don't push,' either. If you just leave it to your body, it really will tell you. And even though they say in the classes about breathing, which American woman really concentrate on a lot, if you just relax and control yourself the baby will come naturally."

Kenly says she feels doctors at birth "are fine, if they're there, keeping their mouths shut. I'm paying them for a service so they can do what I want. It's almost like having an excellent helper there, someone who's experienced and knows what they're doing when I need them. Not someone to tell me what to do."

3. IN A HOUSE ON A WOODED HILL IN A SUBURB, WITH A ROSE-BREASTED GROSBEAK SINGING IN THE WINDOW

David and Joyce are one of those matched couples who say "we got pregnant" and who can finish each other's sentences. As a father, David has been so involved in the births and rearing of his children that the little details of the experience most men never pay attention to—and even Joyce sometimes forgets—David remembers.

They were married later than most couples and had their first child six years after that. David was already comfortably established as an accountant and the couple living in their dream house by the time their first child was born. It is on a woodsy hillside in an attractive Philadelphia suburb, a roomy dwelling designed by

Joyce with children and nature in mind, complete with a rock garden wall and a waterfall leading down to an indoor goldfish pond.

The wait to have a family was not planned but the result of an early inability to conceive. After years of testing and doctor-hopping, the only established medical fact was that David had a low sperm count. "I suspect that vitamin E may have helped correct this," David says. "I had a low sperm count, but after taking vitamin E for some time, it went up. And we got pregnant." The treatment was not prescribed by the many physicians the couple visited. "Oh, come on, we got it from Carlton Fredericks, you know, from listening to the radio," Joyce says. "No, no doctor would ever suggest a thing like that. It makes too much sense."

Another radio program which impressed David and Joyce was one featuring Elisabeth Bing, the childbirth educator. After hearing Bing speak, Joyce decided that if she ever did become pregnant she would surely use the Lamaze method to give birth. "I don't know how we located Mrs. Bing," Joyce says, but after the long-hoped-for pregnancy was confirmed, "we did, and we wrote her and asked if she would refer us to a doctor. I decided, if I'm going to have this baby, I'm so lucky, I'm going to have it exactly right. And I'm not going to have any doctor do me in. And I knew someone who had had a baby and at the last minute the doctors did her in, and I was really very upset by that, and I just decided we were going to have a doctor I could trust." They went to the first one on Mrs. Bing's list. He was matter-of-fact about Lamaze, agreed to breastfeeding on the delivery table, and in answer to a question from Joyce and David, said he did episiotomies "almost 100 percent."

Of the hospitals available where the doctor had privileges, Joyce and David chose one which allowed fathers in the delivery room over one which allowed rooming-in. At the end of what Joyce calls "a delicious labor," the couple spent only two hours in the hospital before the birth of Timothy. Joyce calls the birth "superb," although David insists, "Well, she was elated because she was having her first baby. But the conditions were not good at all." One "condition" was the lithotomy position into which Joyce was strapped on the delivery table, necessitating the use of a forceps to lift the baby's head and guide its exit. It caused a blood clot on the baby's head which remained a long time. Another "condition" was the separation of the new baby from Joyce, which affected her deeply. As she tells it:

"I had asked 'Could I please nurse the baby on the delivery table?' Mrs. Bing had cued us to the necessity of asking, and I thought it was a lovely thing. So I'm lying on my back, right, and they put the baby like that—the doctor did, himself, for about a second and a half."

David explains, "Well, the doctor held him half upside down like this: 'Now, here, nurse. No, he doesn't want to nurse,' and that was the end of that."

"That was exactly what happened," Joyce continues. "Exactly. That was 8:15 so the next feeding quote-unquote would have been at 10. And I was beside myself waiting for that baby because I hadn't really seen him. When ten o'clock arrived the nurse came in and said, 'We're sorry. We can't bring you your baby. His temperature's a little low. We have him in a heated bassinet.' So I didn't question, you know, didn't question. I was absolutely on such a high. I couldn't sleep one wink. I was going over the whole thing. It was so fantastic for me. I was yearning for the baby and going over the whole birth. What an experience! It's a high that's unbelievable. And two o'clock came. And I forget what the reason they gave me then was. The baby was sleeping or something. And they didn't bring the baby then either. And I had four more hours to get through. And for I think the next feeding, at six o'clock, they finally brought him, but the nursing didn't go too well and from here on in things only got worse."

Joyce was signed out of the hospital after four days, although she had paid for eight. For the next three months Joyce experienced a combination of sore, bleeding nipples, a persistent fever, and an infection that she assumes she picked up at the hospital. There was visits with seven doctors in three states, heavy dosages of antibiotics which were ineffective, and lack of correct information on how to establish a good nursing relationship with the baby—who was spending much of his time crying and showing little weight gain. At around the same time David was making phone calls to the Midwest where one knowledgeable doctor had been found. Joyce was recommended to a local doctor who would probably be sympathetic to a mother's wish to breastfeed. The friend who recommended him told Joyce, "He's the kind of guy who'd give you a home delivery." Joyce recalls, "That was the first time I had ever thought of it. But it really just whizzed by my ear. I didn't think any more about it because I wasn't having another baby at that time."

Meanwhile, the midwestern doctor told Joyce to nurse the baby every two hours and prescribed medication over the phone for which the local doctor gave Joyce a written prescription. "And from then on we were going," Joyce says. "That was all we needed to be told. Every other doctor had said, 'Don't nurse until at least three hours have gone by.' Within twenty-four hours I was no longer having any pain, the sore nipples were gone, the baby was no longer unhappy, and everything was roses. It was a long time, but once we learned, it was beautiful. It was really amazing. Because my instincts were so repressed or whatever. I don't know where my instincts were."

"Well," says David, "fortunately, they were rather stubborn. You did have instincts, and they were rather stubborn."

Finally, Joyce says, "I was happy with my baby. And I would have lived happily ever after if I hadn't had another, but I really wanted to." Still concerned about infertility and the fact that she hadn't menstruated by the time Timothy was nine months old, Joyce curtailed nursing somewhat and began menstruating by the time he was a year old. It still took about another nine months to conceive another baby.

Joyce returned to the local doctor to broach the subject of home birth. "By then I think I really felt I wanted it a lot. He was receptive but not eager." He said he would attend Joyce at home, provided the couple agreed to certain provisions. These included having an obstetrical nurse and one other person present and renting a sterile obstetrics pack from the hospital.

For David and Joyce, the sterile pack was typical of what David calls having "a hospital type delivery in the home." Joyce began labor at seven one evening and met the doctor at his office. Her labor promptly stopped. The doctor chided her: "You women don't know anything." Joyce returned home in tears. At home her contractions began again. This time they didn't call the doctor until birth was close at hand. An examination revealed she was fully dilated but the doctor wouldn't let Joyce push. "He was here for quite a while actually," Joyce recalls, "because we went through this whole thing about getting out the sheets" in the sterile pack. "We have a tape of Melanie's delivery," Joyce says, "and it's really amusing. David was really teed off because he had been really into Lamaze at that point and he thought I should be pushing, but the doctor kept saying, 'Don't push because we haven't got the sheets on.' Everything was finally set up and he said I could push and out came Melanie. And I saw the umbilical cord, and I was sure it was a penis. Anyhow it turned out it was a girl. I was thrilled. And I had my baby in my arms. That was the reason I wanted the home delivery, to be able to keep the baby. It wasn't so much for the actual birth experience."

According to David, that experience was "not a satisfactory birth. He gave an episiotomy. Once the doctor came, things didn't go naturally anymore. The doctor was again in control. He doesn't know anything about truly natural deliveries, especially the emotional aspects."

"Or women," Joyce adds.

David and Joyce disagree somewhat on just how the placenta basket routine was put into effect for Melanie's birth. Both knew the advantages of not immediately cutting the umbilical cord, but David had read in a book by Ashley Montagu that the placenta, while still attached to the cord, may be placed in a container high above the level of the baby until the cord drains and dries up. Once it is truly exhausted, usually in about 45 minutes, the scissors which sever it from the baby don't even have to be sterilized. But according to Joyce, "I think David realizes now that fourteen hours is a slight exaggeration." For David, the long wait was "a novelty" and "cute," but for Joyce there are memories of a cold, clammy cord rolling over her belly each time she switched the baby from breast to breast. They cut the cord much sooner with the next two children. (This would not happen if the placenta were placed in a receptacle or on a ladder.)

The third child, a boy named Andrew, was also born at home, attended by the same doctor, and surrounded by a pile of sterile sheets. "But it wasn't the whole multiplicity of them," David says. For the third birth the interference came in the person of a Lamaze teacher who was meeting the doctor's requirement for the obstetrical nurse. A well-meaning friend, this nurse had her own ideas about how things should be done. Predictably, Joyce's labor stopped about five minutes after the Lamaze teacher arrived. Joyce says, "I went up to bed, and David and I cuddled up together. Once we went upstairs and relaxed, the contractions started again. But then whenever the nurse came up, the contractions became erratic or stopped. It was awkward," Joyce says, because it would hurt their friend's feelings if she were told that her good intentions constituted an interference.

"She kept giving interpretations and suggestions," says David. "We should have asked her to wait downstairs until called. When in the childbirth process it's very hard to resist interpretations and suggestions coming from an 'expert.' "

The doctor was finally called, according to Joyce, "a little prematurely, and he kept examining me roughly and just the wrong time. He kept offering me 'a little *Pit*' to speed things up. Again it was a doctor-oriented delivery." This time, though, there was no episiotomy. Joyce's favorite memory of the birth was Timothy's little voice announcing, "It's a boy," his assigned job from his position right under the doctor's knee.

When Andrew was eighteen months old, and Joyce still hadn't resumed menstruating, she met a woman doing a study on suppression of menstruation caused by breastfeeding. Joyce agreed to cooperate with the woman's study by filling out daily records. "We were taking the basal temperature every morning" for months, Joyce says, "and we knew exactly when my first ovulation was. And we conceived. Not that I believe in miracles, but if there ever was one, I think that's one of them, because with my history of not being able to conceive except over a period of months, to conceive on the first ovulation—and I was of such an age." She was forty-one.

"She never did have her period after Andrew's birth," David says.

"So by that time," continues Joyce, "we had learned a lot and really wanted to have a good home delivery. And David was a little more confident of it, I guess, than I was. Because he planned all along to have the baby without a doctor."

Neither David nor Joyce feel that any birth could have turned out better. "This labor was out of this world," Joyce says. "If you could plan a labor, this is the way you'd do it. When I got up in the moring I had a contraction. Just a nice easy contraction, but meaningful, you know. And I said to David, 'Maybe the kids ought to stay home from school today.' And he said, 'Oh, don't be ridiculous. They'll be able to get home in time.' Which was a mistake. Because they were all prepared for this home delivery too."

DAVID: *Anyhow, that was my mistake, sending the kids to school.*

JOYCE: *We cannot talk about regrets.*

DAVID: *Well, we had made arrangements with a friend that if things really got going, the friend would go to school and bring them home. We wanted them all present.*

JOYCE: *But we didn't count on the way things happened or on the fact that they were building sewers and traffic was tied up. But, anyhow, I spent a beautiful morning just having nice contractions, no breathing, mostly daydreaming, you know. It's a beautiful thing. At around eleven o'clock I guess I went down to have a little soup or an egg or something to eat, and on the way up the stairs I said, "David, please call the children." I said it in exactly that tone of voice, and he still didn't do it.*

DAVID: *I said, "Oh, no, no, no, we've got a long time."*

JOYCE: *Yeah, that's exactly what he said. However, at that point, I decided maybe we should call the nurse who had agreed to come— it was a different one this time. So we called her and no answer. And we called her a couple of times. Still no answer, and at that point I decided I had to call the Lamaze teacher who was here last time as our backup. And we called her but she wasn't home either.*

DAVID: *So we were lucky in those respects.*

JOYCE: *So we were stuck there with nobody. Yeah, we were very lucky. And then David called the doctor and said he thought things were happening. And while he was on the phone, I yelled to David: "Things* are *happening." And what was happening was the baby was coming out of the birth canal and was ready to exit. And I was in the throes of a very powerful transition that hit me like a ton of bricks. After this easygoing, beautiful labor, all of a sudden my whole body was taken over. And David had to really slam down the phone on the doctor and rush over. I was on my back on the bed unable to move. And I was even screeching in a panicky way, "I don't know what to do." You know, it was one of those times when you think you're going to forget the whole thing and not have a baby, you know. Yet, it wasn't hurting exactly, it was panic, because I was stretched out in such a way I couldn't move. The baby was right there! I didn't put it all together, you know, in my head at that point. And David said, "Get around vertical" 'cause we had planned definitely that I should be in a vertical position. I had practiced it. You know, we had practiced it over and over, the position I would be in and exactly how I was going to push and everything.*

DAVID: *Or not push.*

JOYCE: *And luckily he helped me. He grabbed my arm and helped me swing around. I got into a vertical position and my body took over. Not like any other experience I have ever had. It was the most beautiful childbirth anyone could ever imagine. It was true birth climax. I didn't push once. I blew and I blew and I did everything I could not to push. And my body just took over and pushed the baby out. And out came this nine-and-a-half pound beauty to the song of a rose-breasted grosbeak sitting on a tree outside the window. And the sun was streaming in the window and I'm looking out into the trees and this bird is there and Stefan is being born. And we didn't have time for anything sterile. We had another hospital pack and we had sheets and towels and newspaper and everything. And we didn't use any of it. He just got born, and I didn't even tear a bit.*

DAVID: *I didn't even wash my hands.*

JOYCE: *And the children arrived about five minutes after that.*

4. A HOME VBAC

Stephanie, an attorney, and Andy, a businessman, live in a small but comfortable house in a residential area of New York City. They have two daughters, Mollie, age 4, born by cesarean, and Meredith, recently homeborn after a long labor. Meredith was born with the assistance of a midwife and with several of Stephanie's friends in attendance. The baby was healthy, but Stephanie, her expanded family in tow, ended up at the hosptial for a few hours anyway. A stubborn placenta had to be removed manually, requiring stitching that the midwife could not perform at home. At the hospital Stephanie was harassed and shortly thereafter investigated for child abuse for having had a home VBAC. The investigation by the Department of Social Services yielded no evidence of child abuse. Stephanie began our interview by recalling the cesarean birth of her first child, Mollie.

I got pregnant with Mollie after about five months of trying. I had been out of law school for a year. I had clerked to a judge for a year and then started my own practice and got pregnant during the same month of August. I had been nauseous for about six weeks but it never occurred to me that I could be pregnant. I was a child then. I see it now I just didn't think *I* could get pregnant. And in my nausea I had such a skewed view of life and feeling that I went to this obstetrician my sister recommened. My sister and I are opposite, like night and day. I mean, she's not into health at all. So I go to this guy in Great Neck and he never once asked me about nutrition. He just gave me pink vitamins; they were disgusting and I felt wrong all along. And I think that feeling wrong all along was one reason that led to a cesarean.

In my sixth month of that first pregnancy somehow I found hospital-based midwives. I had found a Bradley teacher and started taking her class. Maybe she turned me on to going to midwives, I'm not sure. But the midwives I found were wonderful compared to this other fellow, and they were interested in nutrition and stuff like that. But they were still very medical. I didn't know it then but I know it now, just from my instinct of not wanting any of this stuff when I'm pregnant. Birth is not a medical event.

When I went into labor, we were at our country house in East Hampton. Andy wanted to play basketball. He even played basketball the morning that I was due. And I knew then that the next time I was pregnant, I would call the shots and not him. He thought he was so cool; he went to his game, and he told everyone, "My wife's in labor" and all that. And I had a lot of pain, and I just wanted to be home.

We went home and I called my midwife and she said the usual stuff: "You're not far enough along yet" and this and that—very didactic, not something Alice [the midwife of the second birth] said to me which was that if I needed to call, if I was scared, we could talk about why I'm scared. There was no emotional support from my midwives the first time, which was what I expected of them subliminally and never got. I never got anything from them really different from what I got from the doctor except that they were women, physically.

So I was in labor and we were at home and we were panicking. And we were angry. Andy wanted to shower, which I didn't understand. I was in labor forty-eight hours and he needed to have his needs met, but I didn't want to know about that or hear about that. I wanted my needs met. Apparently, we needed someone for him and someone for me.

When I went to the hospital I had brought candy and music. We had this view of how birth was going to be. When I had seen the hosptial for the tour, probably way down deep in my ovaries there was that thought, "You can't give birth here." But I didn't say anything because I didn't see any choice. There was no choice. It was a hospital. There was a bed in it. It was a small bed, too. We have a king-size bed and I thought, "I can't even move in there."

We went to the hospital. I wasn't far enough along, so we went home. I left, and I came back. And we didn't eat, either of us, for fourty-eight hours. When we went back again, I wanted to wear my pink robe. Andy wouldn't hear of it; he thought it was an absurd thing. And I, I thought it was a security blanket, and it was also not getting dressed, it was part of me, bringing me to the hospital. I called it a maternity robe. Also, I had this pain. And there was a sense in all of us of just relieving the pain. It wasn't about having the baby. It was just relieving the pain. I had an epidural for 9 hours, and Mollie had everything, absolutely everything, up to and including a fetal head monitor, that was the *pièce de résistance* for me. And I not only had an epidural, I was asking for a cesarean. And I finally had a cesarean. Andy held her right after she was born. And I nursed her twenty minutes after she was born. I had felt the incision physically because I wasn't anesthetized high enough. The doctor had said, "give me the knife." He didn't call it a scalpel or anything, he just said, "give me the knife."

The hospital was lovely as a nursery because it was very small and cozy and I could just have her all the time. I remember holding her when she was four days old, and I thought I broke her neck because her head was always falling back. I was a new mother. Just as a new pregnant mother. I mean, who knows? I was a little outraged at this notion of men at birth and how wonderful this is. And how they could make it all better. But this is not romance. We have this poster at our summer house—a ballet dancer with pointed toes and leg warmers all worn to pieces. You can think about *Swan Lake* and how beautiful it is, but what does it take to get there? I mean like my second birth, you can think about the birth as joyous and wonderful but I struggled and strained during it. Yet after I got through it and was finished, it was wonderful. I felt that with my first birth also, with Mollie. She made it through. A friend of mine was admiring that I had no bitterness about the cesarean. But I was just grateful for my relationship with Mollie, being with her and nursing her and then being at home with her.

Then she had to go back to the hospital. I had a fever one day, I had the flu and then she had a fever, and I didn't know again. I was a new mother, and they said, "Get her to the hospital. She may have spinal meningitis. Get her there!" And I'm saying, "I

just got through my labor with her, and now we have to go back."
And we did, and she was on IV and she was very cooperative in
some way, so she didn't have to have it in her head. And there I
began to intervene in the hospital. I was beginning to network.
One friend told me my kid didn't have to have an IV if I would
just nurse her more. I asked the doctor about it; rather peacefully,
I said, "Why is she having all this glucose?" And he gave me some
ridiculous reason. He didn't even have the humility to say, "Maybe
you're right." But the next day he just took off the glucose.

"That was my first sense of, "Hey wait a minute. Why are we
going through this stuff?" And then at her six-week check-up the
doctor said, "Now she will have an immunization," and I said, "She
will not." It was a totally emotional decision. I felt she had known
too many needles in her life. At six weeks she would think the
world is about needles, and I just wouldn't have it.

I knew that I wanted to wait a while and really enjoy Mollie
before having another baby which I did.

Meanwhile, a friend mentioned Alice's name and about home
VBACs. I remember when Mollie was about seven months, I went
to a VBAC workshop and I was telling the story and I mentioned
the word "cesarean" and Mollie vomited profusely, to the point
where I got scared and I asked for help. And there was one other
time before that when I mentioned "cesarean" and she vomited
profusely.

A few years later I got pregnant on a weekend and we went to
Washington for the week and we had a ball. When I got home I
called Alice and I had my first appointment. It was the end of
Passover. During Passover, we thought my father had the flu. He
didn't let on how sick he was. But it was the beginning of the end
for him. It was the beginning of a fatal brain tumor. That day that
I had a visit with Alice he was admitted to the hospital. What's
fascinating to me is that Meredith smells like my father.

So I went to Alice, I walked into her home. First of all, it was
her home. This was how it was supposed to be. She was sitting on
a chair or a couch. And she said, "So, tell me what's been going
on." Just talking to her was wonderful. This was a consultation. I
talked about my father, and I cried. Before that I had wanted a
home birth. But when I was learning about my father, when he
was in the hospital, maybe the hospital wasn't so bad if you used
it and were in some control. They weren't doing anything to him

in the hospital. He was just in a bed there. And I said, "Well, maybe that's OK too. Maybe the hosptial is OK."

It was clear that Alice would come with me to the hospital too. I would not go alone with Andy. Andy was relieved with my plan. Now, Andy wasn't for a home birth. He was scared; he wasn't going to tell his mother who was very medical. He used to say up to the end that he'd be at the hospital waiting for us. But I did say to him around the sixth or seventh month: "It doesn't matter what you want; it's my body," which was the cause of some difficulty between us. But ultimately I knew that I couldn't have another cesarean for him. I would hate him. I probably wouldn't divorce him, but I would hate him.

I would see Alice, and she would say, "You're doing fine, and the baby is doing fine." The way that she said it was that we were two individuals. Now, with the midwives the first time they would measure my belly; it was a belly. It was very inhuman and medical. And numbers, who cares about numbers? I hate to get on the scale to check if I'm eating enough. I eat because I'm hungry, so of course I eat enough. I eat well, and that's enough.

The second time it was very spiritual all along. My father was dying. At the beginning of my pregnancy I was nauseous and I wasn't eating. So my friends would cook for me. And that eating, that feeding of the child within, was more valuable than 40 hundred calories. I could relate to Alice with that. Alice is a very spiritual metaphysical woman, which was what I needed.

When I saw Alice I would discuss whatever it was that was pertinent then. It was wonderful. We'd talk about my father. We'd talk about his living and dying. What was great about Alice was she would talk about herself. It was different from a therapist relationship because she was a human being sharing her life. I was very inspired about the fact that she had five kids, that she had births at home, and that she was so imperfect; that's what I loved about her—that she was human. She wasn't inapproachable.

When I would visit my father I just felt that there was a window in my belly and Meredith was looking out at my father. My father also got well in the middle. He had gone to Germany for one of those treatments. He was just here, regular, and it was wild. Also, as part of my discussions with Alice, I was able to let him go when he got sick again. I encouraged my family to let him die. When we were contemplating alternatives; it was just unrealistic to go every other month to Germany, for him to stay well, and to bring

him in and out of that. It was the letting go. My father was a man
of his convictions. He believed in alternatives, and he wouldn't let
them do radiation. And ultimately with Mollie's birth I suppose it
was the same thing. I had changed midwives but they weren't
nearly as resourceful as I had hoped they would be. And just going
to the hospital was wrong. So it seemed to follow that I would have
the cesarean. Just going the medical route, that whole thing.

Along the way with Alice I decided that I would have a home
birth. I had to make a decision about that because there were
certain things I would have to buy. Just buying the things and
having them here was another very good reality, that I could do
this, that I could prepare in my own home for this birth.

Labor was wonderful. I labor long. I labored forty-eight hours
with Mollie, and I labored thirty-six hours with Meredith.

Late on a Monday evening I felt pinchy cramps, and it was fun.
I was saying, "Come, come, you can come now." In fact, that day
I had seen Alice, two days after my due date. And she said, "You
can have this baby, Stephanie, it's OK." Cause I thought I would
be three weeks late. It was interesting because I had gone into
labor with Mollie by scared induction. They threatened me with
what they called a stress test. They didn't even call it a nonstress
test. I had to be at the hospital. And I didn't even want to know
what it was about. That again meant something was wrong. They
were going to do it two days after my due date. But the way Alice
coaxed me gently into labor if I chose was a whole different thing.
It was the same message but a different way of giving it.

My back-up doctor had said, "Well, you know, if you're at 2
centimeters for two days, I'm going to have to induce you with
Pitocin." He thought this was wonderful because he wasn't doing
another cesarean. He was very skeptical about me because I was
a lawyer. I had told him I would sign a release form. And he said
to me, "you should know as a lawyer that releases don't hold." I
mean what kind of a society is it if releases don't hold, if things
don't matter? I'm entitled to do what I want with my body. I had
worked out things with him if I had to go to the hospital because
my midwife and my VBAC teacher had gently pushed me in that
direction. They said "YOU have to deal with this." At one point
the back-up doctor said to me, "Are you sure you want to work
with me?" My answer was, "I want you to know it's not you. I don't
like medicine. I don't like hospitals. It's not you."

Now, I'm in labor. And my plan for the next day was to walk.

My plan that day was to take Mollie for Japanese food and then to the library. And I did, carrying the stroller on the bus and everything. And I was in labor. And what I did was I would blow out. Not Lamaze blow out but blow it out instead of keeping it in, like I did with Mollie. One of the healing things I had at the VBAC class was the notion of the tight squeeze. And at the restaurant Mollie would blow out with me. So it was a real pleasure to labor with Mollie again.

At home, I labored at the table. And I was massaging my back. I had no inkling that I could do that with Mollie. I guess I had a sense that I had to be rescued. This notion of men with their wives in labor meant to me that my husband would take away the pain. That was why in this birth Alice couldn't even massage my perineum. "As long as you're going to do that," I thought, "then take the baby."

While I was at the table, Andy called up; he was with a client in the city. He had wanted me to use his beeper but I hadn't even learned the number. If it happened so fast I would do it myself, and if it didn't happen so fast then he would get home in time. He wasn't going to rescue me, and he wasn't going to be able to do anything much for me, so I didn't need him. I used to envision my labor happening upstairs alone while all the other people stayed on the main floor. I knew that nobody could do it for me. But I didn't know it was going to be this painful. I had totally forgotten. I don't even know if it was that painful, as much as I was scared.

Andy came home, and he had this macho attitude about who we should call first. But I've also been able to listen to him, which I've learned to do. We had it rough during the pregnancy. I didn't trust him, and I needed only to rely on me. I felt that he had deceived me because he had gone to the other side during Mollie's birth; he had gone the medical route. Even though I don't agree with Andy a lot of times I should just listen. That's all I do is listen.

Birthing at home by myself without intervention was like a drug. I don't know a lot of what happened. During the strong labor later in my room I knew just what I needed and everything else was just not there, just did not exist. I just slept between contractions. I actually slept! I was only interested in myself, in a selfish, good way. I just need what I need. It was totally primal.

Then it was later at night. And Alice came. One of my friends came and said I had to go see the moon. I needed to go outside, to know that the world was bigger than me. I need physicality. I have to see that the world is greater than me, that this happens, and it has happened before, and it will happen again. When I went out I remember I wore my father's wool hat. I just use my father in a very positive way. I just use all he's given me. And that's what I go on now, that he's given me so much.

Possibly the next baby I would gently push. I didn't need to push Meredith out. Not that she wasn't ready to be born, but I could have pushed her. However, notwithstanding that, I do respect Alice's professional decision to make me push, because until that baby was out, I did not know that I would have a VBAC; and I think it was important for me to know that I was going to have a VBAC. And in order to do that she needed to push me to push.

I could never have done a natural birth in the hospital, not with this birth. And now I know too that when some people say natural, they've had epidurals. And they call that natural. I'm not judging that, but mine was like an animal. I had to give birth, I had to do it wild, and it was just different.

I remember screaming so loud and saying, "I'm screaming louder than it hurts." I guess it did hurt. But I feel like it hurt because I was being forced to push. And all this happened because I was at home. Whatever happened happened because I was at home. Having tea, having people here when I needed them; when I didn't need them they were gone. The lights were low, it was my own bed. I was very much like an animal.

When I was hanging on my door I thought I was a monkey in Africa. I thought birth was sexual and private, and I wanted to be alone. I didn't want anyone to watch. But it was fun seeing my friends hanging out here. They were sitting around the table talking, talking about me, talking about things. It was just real neat that this was all happening.

The hospital was very much a part of Meredith's birth. I'm just glad it was I and not she who had to go. The stitches didn't take. Alice said it was because I had to go to the hospital for other reasons, because I had to deal with the hosptial. It has to be the antidote to Mollie's birth. Mollie's birth had been so laden with interventions that I couldn't have a panacea birth with Meredith. That would have been too much of a gift, too much of a miracle to have a wonderful, easy birth. I needed to grapple with the past, which I did. I got over a lot of the bad things that were in Mollie's birth.

After they sutured me, they wanted to explore my uterus and I said, "You will not." They wanted to see if I was ruptured; but they'll rupture me first.

I often say to Alice, "Thank you." Not thank you for helping me give birth—I did it—but I needed her support. I know that that was vital. She said, "All that I did was give you the space to birth." Which is very humble. But it's ironic in its way that in our society you don't very often get that space. It's weird that you even need that space. Why do people think they can control whether I give birth in the home or not? That we've had a whole birth in this house effected the karma of this house. We weren't angry at the first cesarean. It just had to be that way. And I labor slowly because I just do things slowly. I'm always late. I do things slow.

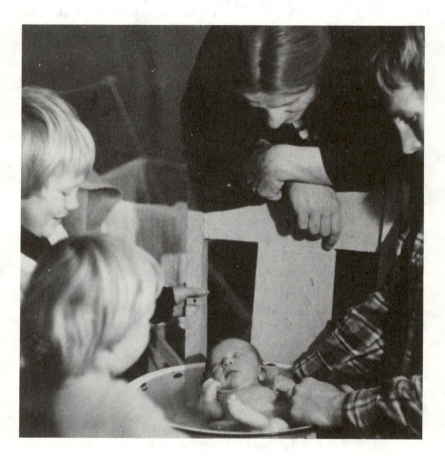

Byron Greatorex photograph

Postscript

W e are at a real turning point in the sequence of events of childbirth reform in this country. Home birth, which was the nineteenth-century norm, was replaced by the middle of this century by routine and virtually unquestioning compliance with hospital birth. Now women want to swing the pendulum back. When the first edition of this book was published in the late '70s, their activities were secretive and virtually unnoticed. Now, quickly, it is like an all-out war.

The medical profession has noticed that we are out here and is using aggressive tactics—be they widespread lies, rewriting of laws or hospital privilege policies, or instigating arrests—to fight back. A home birth population of less than 5 percent nationally, although growing, should not be a threat. We are not, on the face of it, but there are larger issues here, issues like control and economics. Who should control a woman's reproduction? The medical profession, society at large, or each individual mother? And what of economics? How do rising malpractice insurance rates and increased demand for midwife services affect obstetrics as a profession?

Lost in the complexity of these larger issues is that individual mother and baby who need prenatal care now for a birth this year. What is safest, healthiest, and most satisfying for them? The delegates to the largest international conference on home birth in October 1987 had their answer, and the delegates to the ACOG convention had theirs. But that mother and baby need their answers now.

In countries where home birth is tolerated, even supported, good prenatal care is available to all women, regardless of the intended place of birth. And women with complications arising at a home birth are welcomed to the hospital, without punishment, because that is the place that can help them best now.

Perhaps it would be prudent to take local (United States) politics out of a universal issue like birth and listen to the recommendations of the Joint Interregional Conference on Appropriate Technolgy for Birth (held in Brazil, April 1985) which recommended that:

> The whole community should be informed about the various procedures in birth care, to enable each woman to choose the type of birth care she prefers.
>
> Informal perinatal care systems (including traditional birth attendants), where they exist, must coexist with the official birth care system, and collaboration between them must be maintained for the benefit of the mother. Such relations, when established in parallel with no concept of superiority of one system over the other, can be highly effective.
>
> Obstetric care services that have critical attitudes towards technology and that have adopted an attitude of respect for the emotional, psychological, and social aspects of birth care should be identified. Such services should be encouraged, and the processes that have led them to their position must be studied so that they can be used as models to foster similar attitudes in other centers and to influence obstetrical views nationwide.

Isn't it about time?

Chapter Notes

Chapter 3

1. Dr. Robert Mendelsohn, personal communication.

2. Metropolitan Life Insurance Company, "Report on the Frontier Nursing Service of Hayden, Kentucky," May 9, 1932. See also H. Browne and G. Isaacs, "The Frontier Nursing Service, "*American Journal of Obstetrics and Gynecology* 124 (1976): 14–17, and "Summary of First 10,000 Confinement Records of the Frontier Nursing Service," *Quarterly Bulletin of Frontier Nursing Service* 33 (Spring 1958): 45–55.

3. New York Academy of Medicine, *Maternal Mortality in New York City* (New York: The Commonwealth Fund, 1933).

4. Myron E. Wegman, "Annual Summary of Vital Statistics," *Pediatrics* 78 (Dec. 1986): 983–94.

5. Thomas Cianfrani, *A Short History of Obstetrics and Gynecolocy* (Springfield, Ill.: Charles C. Thomas, 1960), p. 403.

6. Raven Lang, *The Birth Book* (Ben Lomond, Calif.: Genesis Press, 1972).

7. Lester Dessez Hazell, *Birth Goes Home* (Seattle: Catalyst, 1974).

8. Diana Korte and Roberta Scaer, *A Good Birth, A Safe Birth* (New York: Bantam, 1984).

9. C. Burnett el al., "Home Delivery and Neonatal Mortality in North Carolina," *Journal of the American Medical Association* 244 (1980): 2741–45; M. Hinds et al., "Neonatal Outcome in Planned *vs.* Unplanned

Out-of-Hospital Births in Kentucky," *Journal of the American Medical Association* 253 (1985): 1578–82; and D. Sullivan and R. Beeman, "Four Years' Experience with Home Birth by Licensed Midwives in Arizona," *Journal of the American Public Health Association* 73 (1983): 641–45.

10. American College of Obstetricians and Gynecologists, "Health Department Data Show Danger of Home Births" (Jan. 4, 1978).

Chapter 4

1. R. Sosa et al., "The Effect of a Supportive Companion on Perinatal Problems, Length of Labor and Mother-Infant Interaction," *New England Journal of Medicine* 303 (1980): 597–600.

2. D. Liebeskind et al., "Morphological Changes in the Surface Characteristics of Cultured Cells After Exposure to Diagnostic Ultrasound," *Radiology* 138 (1981): 419–23, and D. Liebeskind et al., "Diagnostic Ultrasound: Time Lapse and Transmission Electron Microscope Studies in Cells Insonated in Vitro," *British Journal of Cancer* (Supplement V) 45 (1982): 176–86.

3. Doris Haire, "The Cultural Unwarping of Childbirth: How Can It Be Accomplished?" in Stewart and Stewart, *21st Century Obstetrics Now!* 2nd ed. (Chapel Hill, N. C.: NAPSAC, 1977), pp. 567–84.

4. Jay Hathaway, "Controversy in Ultrasound," *ABCC News* 3(1983): 2.

5. Albert Haverkamp et al., "The Evaluation of Continuous Fetal Heart Rate Monitoring in High-Risk Pregnancy," *American Journal of Obstetrics and Gynecology* 125 (1976): 310–17.

6. H. David Banta and Stephen B. Thacker, "Costs and Benefits of Electronic Fetal Monitoring: A Review of the Literature," Office of Health Research, Statistics, and Technology, U. S. Department of Health, Education, and Welfare, April 1979.

7. K. J. Levano et al., "A Prospective Comparison of Selective and Universal Electronic Fetal Monitoring in 34,995 Pregnancies," *New England Journal of Medicine* 315 (1986): 615–19.

8. Paul Placek, "The Cesarean Future," *American Demographics* (Sept. 1987).

9. J. R. Evrard and E. M. Gold, "Cesarean Section and Maternal Mortality in Rhode Island," *Obstetrics and Gynecology* 50 (1977): 594.

10. Kieran O'Driscoll and Michael Foley, "Correlation of Decrease in Perinatal Mortality and Increase in Cesarean Section Rates," *Obstetrics and Gynecology* 61 (1983): 1–5.

11. Shirley Hutchcroft et al., "Late Results of Cesarean and Vaginal Delivery in Cases of Breech Presentation," *Canadian Medical Association Journal* 125 (1981): 726–30.

12. For a fuller discussion of VBAC, see Lynn Baptisti Richards, *The Vaginal Birth After Cesarean (VBAC) Experience* (S. Hadley, Mass.; Bergin & Garvey, 1987).

13. Susan G. Doering, "Unnecessary Cesareans: Doctor's Choice, Patient's Dilemma," in Stewart and Stewart, *Compulsory Hospitalization or Freedom of Choice in Childbirth,* I (Marble Hill, Mo.: NAPSAC, 1979).

Chapter 5

1. Pat Carter, *Come Gently, Sweet Lucina* (Titusville, Fla.: Patricia Cloyd Carter, 1957).

2. John S. Miller, "Parents and Professionals: Partners in Childbirth," presentation at ICEA Sixth Biennial Convention, April 1970.

3. Ina May Gaskin, "MANA Formed," *The Practicing Midwife* 1 (Summer 1982): 5.

4. The American College of Nurse-Midwives, The American College of Obstetricians and Gynecologists, and The Nurses Association of The American College of Obstetricians and Gynecologists, "Joint Statement on Maternity Care," 1971.

Chapter 6

1. Mayer Eisenstein, "Homebirths and the Physician," in Stewart and Stewart, *Safe Alternatives in Childbirth* (Chapel Hill, N. C.: NAPSAC, 1976), pp. 67–71.

2. Gail Sforza Brewer, with Tom Brewer, *What Every Pregnant Woman Should Know: The Truth About Diets and Drugs in Pregnancy* (New York: Random House, 1977), and Agnes C. Higgins, "Nutritional Status and the Outcome of Pregnancy," *Journal of the Canadian Dietetic Association* 37(1976): 17.

3. David E. Barrett, "An Approach to the Conceptualization and Assessment of Social-Emotional Functioning in Studying Nutrition-Behavior Relationships," *American Journal of Clinical Nutrition (5 Supplement)* 5(1982): 1222–27, and Nancy Klein et al., "Preschool Performance of Children with Normal Intelligence Who Were Very-Low-Birth-Weight Infants," *Pediatrics* 75 (1985): 531–37.

4. National Center for Health Statistics, Community Nutrition Institute (Washington, D. C.), "Pregnant Mothers Gaining Less Weight," *CNI News,* Sept. 4, 1986, p. 6.

5. "A Solid Investment in Healthier Babies," *Newsday* (Long Island) editorial, Feb. 9, 1986.

6. Gail Sforza Brewer. with Tom Brewer, *The Brewer Medical Diet for Normal and High-Risk Pregnancy* (New York: Simon & Schuster, 1983).

7. "Medical Research Council Working Party on Amniocentesis," *British Journal of Obstetrics and Gynaecology* 85 (1978): 1661–62.

8. Sarah Arneson, "Automobile Seat Belt Practices of Pregnant Woman," *Journal of Obstetrics, Gynecologic, and Neonatal Nursing* 4 (July-Aug. 1986): 339–44.

9. Arthur D. Colman and Libby Lee Colman, *Pregnancy: The Psychological Experience* (New York: Herder & Herder, 1971).

Chapter 7

1. Dorothy Brooten et al., "A Randomized Clinical Trial of Early Hospital Discharge and Home Follow-Up of Very-Low-Birth-Weight Infants," *New England Journal of Medicine* (1986): 931–39.

2. Sheila Kitzinger, "Episiotomy: Physical and Emotional Aspects," London: National Childbirth Trust, 1981.

3. Frederick Leboyer, *Birth Without Violence* (New York: Knopf, 1975).

Chapter 8

1. Marshall H. Klaus and John H. Kennell, *Maternal-Infant Bonding: The Impact of Early Separation or Loss on Family Development* (St. Louis: C. V. Mosby, 1976).

2. Ashley Montagu, *Touching: The Human Significance of the Skin,* 3rd ed. (New York: Harper & Row, 1987).

3. Rene Spitz, *The First Year of Life: A Psychosomatic Study of Normal and Deviant Development of Object Relations* (New York: International Universities Press, 1965).

4. Adelle Davis, *Let's Have Healthy Children* (New York: New American Library, 1972).

Chapter 9

1. "Hospitals Can Be Dangerous to Your Health," *Alternatives* (newsletter of the Health Alternatives Legal Foundation, Dothan, Ala.), Sept. 1986.

2. To request a copy, send a stamped, self-addressed envelope to the AHA at 840 Lake Shore Drive, Chicago, Ill. 60611.

3. George J. Annas, *The Rights of Hospital Patients* (New York: Avon, 1975).

4. *A Summary Report* (ICP/MCH 102/mo2[S], 0175V, 10 June 1985) in English may be requested from: World Health Organization, U. N. Plaza, New York, N. Y. 10017.

5. "Obstetric, Gynecologic, and Neonatal Nursing Functions and Standards" may be ordered from: The Nurses Association of The American College of Obstetricians and Gynecologists, 1 East Wacker Dr., Suite 2000, Chicago, Ill. 60601. "Standards of Hospital Care for Newborns" is available from: The American Academy of Pediatrics, 141 Northwest Point Rd., P. O. Box 927, Elk Grove Village, Ill. 60007.

Suggestions for Further Reading

Annas, G. J. *The Rights of Hospital Patients*. New York: Avon Books, 1975.

Arms, S. *Immaculate Deception*. So. Hadley, Ma.: Bergin & Garvey, 1975.

Bean, C. *Labor & Delivery: An Observer's Diary*. Garden City, N.Y.: Doubelday, 1977.

———. *Methods of Childbirth*. Garden City, N.Y.: Doubleday, 1974.

Bradley, R. *Husband-Coached Childbirth*. New York: Harper & Row, 1974.

Brewer, G. S. *The Pregnancy-After-30 Workbook*. Emmaus, Pa.: Rodale, 1978.

———.*What Every Pregnant Woman Should Know: The Truth about Diet & Drugs in Pregnancy*. New York: Random House, 1977.

Elkins, V. H. *The Rights of the Pregnant Parent*. New York: Schocken, 1980.

Gaskin, I. M. *Spiritual Midwifery*. Summertown, Tenn.: The Book Publishing Co., 1975.

Hartman, R. *Exercises for True Natural Childbirth*. New York: Harper & Row, 1975.

Jacobson, E. *How to Relax & Have Your Baby*. New York: McGraw-Hill, 1965.

Klaus, M., & J. Kennell. *Maternal-Infant Bonding*. St. Louis: C.V. Mosby, 1976.

Korte, D., and R. Scaer. *A Good Birth, A Safe Birth*. New York: Bantam, 1984.

Leavitt, J. W. *Brought to Bed: Childbearing in America 1750–1950*. New York: Oxford University Press, 1986.

Nilsson, L. *A Child Is Born*. New York: Delacorte, 1979.

Noble, E. *Essential Exercises for the Childbearing Year*. Boston: Houghton Mifflin, 1976.

Rooks, J., and J. E. Haas. *Nurse-Midwifery in America*. Washington, D.C.: The American College of Nurse-Midwifery Foundation, 1986.

Stewart & Stewart, eds. *The Childbirth Activist's Handbook*. Marble Hill, Mo.: NAPSAC Reproductions, 1983.

The Womanly Art of Breastfeeding. Franklin Park, Ill.: La Leche League International, 1987.

Wallerstein, E. *Circumcision: An American Health Fallacy*. New York: Springer, 1980.

Ward, C., and F. Ward. *The Home Birth Book*. Washington, D.C.: Inscape, 1976.

Williams, P. *Nourishing Your Unborn Child.* New York: Avon, 1974.

Equipment for Home Birth

M ost of the equipment you need for a home birth is right on your own person: a well-nourished body with functioning parts, and a good attitude. Most other things can easily be found in the average home or can be safely substituted: if you don't have receiving blankets for wrapping the baby, towels, sheets, or an adult blanket will keep her warm, too. But if you are the organized type who is anxious to fill the waiting cradle with something in the meantime, here are some suggestions.

> Plastic mattress cover (a shower curtain will do)
> Old clean sheets for the birth
> Clean sheets for after the birth (this doesn't mean you have to give birth on a bed)
> Newspapers (especially if you're not giving birth on a bed)
> Old clean bath towels, face towels, wash cloths, receiving blankets (several of each)
> Lots of pillows
> Lots of food, especially healthy liquids like juices, raspberry leaf tea, and energy drinks like Third Wind

Simple clean clothes for the new baby to wear after birth, in-
cluding a hat (Some midwives like these wrapped in foil to be
warmed in a slow oven at the end of labor) and diapers
Pot for boiling water
Pot or bowl to hold placenta
Nightgowns suitable for breastfeeding
Sanitary napkins and belt
Disposable bed pads

If you will be acting as baby catchers yourselves, there are several items of professional equipment you may wish to purchase,
such as a fetoscope for auscultating the baby's heart tones and
clamps for cutting the umbilical cord (remember, boiled shoelaces
do as well). Part of the problem in acquiring this equipment is that
one can't just walk into any drug store or department store baby
section and purchase a fetoscope. Sometimes one can be borrowed
from a childbirth educator who has assisted at labors, and in some
states birthing supplies may be ordered by mail through a cata-
logue. An example of such a mail order house is:

Cascade Birthing
P. O. Box 12203
Salem, Ore. 97309
(503) 378–7545.

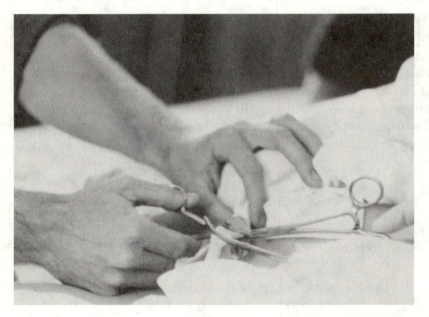

Byron Greatorex photograph

Nutrition/Diet

There are probably as many nutritional styles and diet plans as there are earthly foods fit for human consumption. What is a natural food to one person, like beans, might not be eaten by another unless they were grown in a particular soil and environment. And one type of vegetarian may eat chicken and fish but eliminate red meat while another will eat none of those, nor milk and eggs either. (Some vegetarians may find they want to add some foods to their pregnancy diet that they don't ordinarily eat.) Rather than join the debate over which diet style is best (and feasible), let me stress the importance of *enough* food during pregnancy to grow a big, healthy, full-term baby, and also to grow a strong uterus and keep the mother's body in excellent working order. For most women this means a diet of 100 grams of protein daily from meat, dairy, and/or beans, with a lot of fresh vegetables and fruits and whole grains. To that end I present first an example of a daily pregnancy diet (portion sizes are flexible since you should eat to taste and drink to thirst in pregnancy) and then a list of common protein-containing foods with the number of grams of protein for each. (Remember, salt is a necessary nutrient in pregnancy.)

One Day's Sample Menu

Breakfast	2 eggs
	2 slices whole wheat toast with butter
	glass of orange juice
	glass of milk
Morning snack	cup of plain yogurt over sliced banana, sprinkled with wheat germ
Lunch	tuna fish salad with fresh greens
	corn muffin
	glass of milk
Afternoon snack	nuts, seeds, and raisins mixture
Supper	bowl of lentil soup
	1/4 chicken
	broccoli
	sweet potato
	glass of milk
Bedtime snack (especially if you are breastfeeding a toddler, playing tennis daily, or have the flu)	peanut butter sandwich on whole-grain bread
	glass of milk

Protein Value of Common Foods, in Grams

Grains

bread, 2-inch slice	2
pancake, 4-inch diam.	2
waffle, 5-inch diam.	5
muffin, average	3
dry cereal, commercial, 1 cup	2–4
spaghetti, cooked, 1 cup	7
cake, 1 average slice	4
oatmeal cookie, 4 inch diam.	2
fruit pie, 1 average slice	4
popcorn, 2 cups	3
brown rice, 1/3 cup	5

Dairy

milk, all types; yogurt, 1 cup	8
cheddar cheese, 1/4 inch slice	7
cottage cheese, 1/2 cup	22
cream cheese, 2 Tbs.	3

vanilla ice cream, 1/2 cup	3
pudding, 1/2 cup	4
egg	6

Meat and Fish

flounder or sole, 4 oz.	17
haddock or halibut, average fillet	22
salmon, average fillet	20
tuna, 7 oz. can	35
shrimp, 5 large	13
beef, average serving, or 1 large hamburger	20–25
frankfurter, 1 average	7
liver, average slice or 1 large chicken liver	8
pork chop, 1 medium	16
veal cutlet, 3 oz.	22
chicken, 1/4	22
turkey, 1 average slice	10

Fruit

avocado	4
banana, large	2
cantalope, large	4
grapefruit, large	3
figs, 4	2
orange, large	2
raisins, 1 cup	4
watermelon, average slice	3

(most other fruits and fruit juices, less than 1 gm. per serving)

Nuts and Seeds

peanut butter, 1 Tb.	4
peanuts, 1 cup	30
almonds, 1 cup	21
cashews, 1 cup	19
sunflower seeds, hulled, 1/2 cup	13
walnuts, 1 cup	17

Vegetables

navy beans, cooked, 1 cup	17
kidney beans, cooked, 1 cup	11
lentils, dry, 1/3 cup	17
tofu, 4 oz.	9
soybean sprouts, 4 oz.	7
broccoli, cooked, 1 cup	5
brussel sprouts, 5	3
lettuce wedge, small	1

mushrooms, 3 large	2
peas, cooked, 1/2 cup	3
potato	2–3
spinach, 1/2 cup	3
tomato, small	1

Helpful Contacts

A number of the childbirth groups mentioned in this book may be helpful to you. Some have classes or lists of birth attendants available in various parts of the country. Some of these organizations are managed by volunteers on a limited budget, so kindly enclose a stamped, self-addressed envelope when requesting a reply. Following are the names and addresses:

American Academy of Husband-Coached Childbirth
[Bradley method]
P. O. Box 5224
Sherman Oaks, Calif. 91413

American Foundation for Maternal and Child Health
30 Beekman Place
New York, N. Y. 10022

American Society for Psychoprophylaxis
in Obstetrics (ASPO)
[Lamaze method]
1411 K Street, N. W.
Washington, D. C. 20005

Cesarean Prevention Movement
P. O. Box 152
Syracuse, N. Y. 13210

Health Alternatives Legal Foundation
105 North Foster Street
Dothan, Ala. 36302

Informed Birth & Parenting
P. O. Box 3675
Ann Arbor, Mich. 48106

International Association of Parents and Professionals
for Safe Alternatives in Childbirth (NAPSAC)
Rt. 1, Box 646
Marble Hill, Mo. 63764

International Childbirth Education Association (ICEA)
P. O. Box 20048
Minneapolis, Minn. 55420

La Leche International [breastfeeding]
9616 Minneapolis Avenue
Franklin Park, Ill. 60131

Metropolitan New York Childbirth Education Association
[cooperative childbirth]
P. O. Box 2036
New York, N. Y. 10185

Midwives Alliance of North America (MANA)
P. O. Box 5337
Cheyenne, Wyo. 82003

The New Nativity
P. O. Box 6223
Leawood, Kan. 66206

INDEX